Acupuncture Is Like Noodles

Acupuncture Is Like Noodles

the Little Red (Cook)Book of Working Class Acupuncture

Lisa Rohleder,
Skip Van Meter,
Moses Cooper,
Matthew Gulbransen,
Joseph Goldfedder,
JOhn Vella

Copyright 2009 Working Class Acupuncture

Lisa Rohleder, Skip Van Meter, Moses Cooper, Matthew Gulbransen, Joseph Goldfedder, John Vella

All rights reserved

www.workingclassacupuncture.org

Fist Logo: Choon-Soo Paek
Artwork: Moses Cooper
Book Design & Editing: Matthew Gulbransen

Printed in Portland, Oregon

First Edition

This book is dedicated to all of the patients of the community acupuncture movement (without whom there would be no movement), and especially to Michael McCoy, without whom there would be no Community Acupuncture Network.

Thank You

Your purchase of this book not only helps Working Class Acupuncture to create more affordable acupuncture clinics in Oregon, it helps the community acupuncture movement to spread nationally and internationally.

Disclaimer

This book is intended to provide only general, non-specific information about the practice of community acupuncture within the context of the American health care system. It is meant as an educational reference for acupuncturists and acupuncture students interested in setting up clinics that use the community acupuncture business model, and as a broad overview for interested patients and laypeople.

The level of detail contained in this book should not lead anyone to interpret it as a how-to manual; we have included a lot of detail about acupuncture because recent studies suggest that only about 1% of the American population has tried acupuncture, and the purpose of this book is simply to give people who are unfamiliar with acupuncture a context for our discussion. The acupuncture treatment suggestions and protocols in this book should be used by qualified practitioners only. The authors accept no responsibility for the results of use or misuse of the information contained in this book, or for any errors or omissions in this information; we are simply trying to explain what we do, why we do it, and what we believe, because so many people keep asking us. What we do and what we believe are not necessarily applicable to your particular situation, so please do not apply anything that you read here uncritically. We trust you to have some common sense.

The views expressed in this book are solely those of Working Class Acupuncture and its employees, and do not necessarily represent those of any other community acupuncturists or of the nonprofit Community Acupuncture Network. The fact that this book is helping to raise funds for CAN does not oblige CAN or any of its members to agree with WCA. We trust you all to think for yourselves.

Contents

Introduction 1
   No, it's a revolution. Albeit a very peaceful one. 3
   But what does acupuncture have to do with revolution? 3
   Congratulations, you've just imagined the
   community acupuncture movement! .4

Part One: Acupuncture is Like Noodles 7
   Just as nobody knows where acupuncture originated,
   nobody really knows why it works. .10
   Acupuncture nourishes the body by helping it to relax. 11
   About Acupuncture in America. 11
   What good to anyone is a single, overpriced noodle? 12
   The Social Responsibility of Noodles. 13
   Making Simple Noodles: the Kitchen
   and the Dining Room. 16
   Class and Noodles. 17
   Two Types of Noodles. 20
   Acupuncturists: Use Your Noodles!. 22

Part Two: Welcome to Our Kitchen 25
   Thank You, Michael Pollan. 29
   Ingredients and Recipes 32
   But First: Thank You, NADA 32
   Oh, If Only We Ruled the World:
   Acupuncture Education 34
   Points/Ingredients. 36
   How We Treat Pain. 49
   How We Treat Conditions Other Than Pain. 49

Unilateral/Bilateral 51
Okay, Now We Will Explain How We Treat Pain. 51
Needling In Clusters 53
A Few Pain Recipes, with Explanations. 53
Cooking: Get the Needles in the Patients with a
Minimum of Fuss and Then Leave Them In as
Long as They Want. And Repeat. 56
How Our Treatment Room Looks and Why. 59

Part Three: Welcome to Our Dining Room (and Our Systems) 63
Our Basic Systems. 67
Why We Love Our Systems .73
Systems and Relationships. 76
Money Systems 78
Social Business, Money, and Self Respect 81

Part Four: Reflections on the Kitchen and the Dining Room, from Several Different Angles 85
What's the Point of the Community Acupuncture
Business Model? By Skip. 87
Just the Acupuncture Part By John 95
Tales from the Trenches: My Paradigm Shift from
TCM to Community Acupuncture by Moses 96
Slowing Down to Speed Up by Matthew 102
OK, I've Built It. Now Where the Heck Are They?
Some Thoughts on Growing a Patient Base by Lisa 105
Practice, Practice, Practice by Moses 110
If I Were Going to Start My Own
Acupuncture School by Joseph. 113

Part Five: Health Care Reform and Noodles. 115
Nobody Owns Acupuncture:
Licensing, Classism, and Turf Warfare 119
We feel a need to radically redefine
this particular discourse. 121
Beyond Professionalism, Toward Usefulness 121
What the Future Could Look Like. 123
Community Acupuncture IS Health Care Reform 125

Appendix A: Handling Needles. 127
Opening the Needle Pack 127
Removing the Needle 128
Loading the Guide Tube 128
Holding the Needle Ready .129

    Placing the Needle 129
    Inserting the Needle 130
    Removing the Guide Tube 130
    Adjusting the Needle. 131
Appendix B: Patient Welcome Letter **133**
    Welcome to Our Community! 133
    What is different about the WCA clinic?. 133
    Our Commitment to You 134
    What We Need From You 135
Notes **139**
    Introduction 139
    Part One: Acupuncture is Like Noodles 139
    Part Two: Welcome to Our Kitchen 139
    Part Three: Welcome to Our Dining Room 140
Bibliography **141**

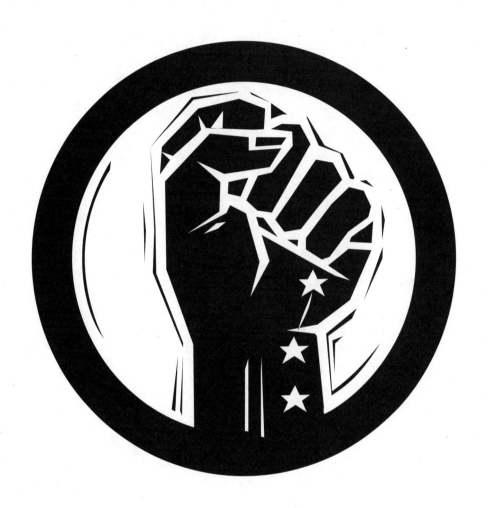

Introduction

Why, all over America, is there suddenly a profusion of dimly lit rooms full of second-hand recliners, filled with peacefully dozing people – people of all ages, races, backgrounds, and occupations, all napping together? And why, if you look closely, do all of those people have very tiny needles sticking out of their hands and feet and heads? What is this, some kind of a cult?

No, it's a revolution. Albeit a very peaceful one.[1]

The purpose of this book is to explain, and also to advance, the community acupuncture movement. It is meant as a response to many of the questions that different people have asked us over the last couple of years -- patients, acupuncturists and acupuncture students, as well as journalists, educators, and plenty of folks who are simply curious about what we call, affectionately, the revolution.

But what does acupuncture have to do with revolution?

Imagine what would happen if a pharmaceutical company announced that it had invented a drug which could effectively treat practically everything that could go wrong with a person. The short list would include asthma, arthritis, indigestion, PMS, sinusitis, insomnia, fibromyalgia, hot flashes, high blood pressure, infertility, constipation, the side effects of chemotherapy, and the common cold, not to mention every conceivable variety of pain. And imagine that not only can this drug address all of these problems, but all of its "side effects" are positive: it has stress-reducing and mood-elevating properties, and in fact is so relaxing that some people who have nothing really wrong with them like to use it on a regular basis, just because they enjoy it so much. And yet it isn't addictive, and there's no way to overdose on it. Think about the potential market for such a drug -- and how it would challenge our assumptions about how medicine works.

Now imagine that this drug isn't a drug, but a practice so old that it cannot be patented or claimed by anyone.

A practice that requires almost no materials and potentially costs almost nothing.

In a country that is not only in the midst of a health care crisis due to skyrocketing costs, but also sunk in the worst recession in memory.

See where we're going with this?

But wait -- imagine that unfortunately this practice that should cost almost nothing and should be available to virtually everybody has somehow become so expensive that almost nobody can even afford to try it. And to add insult to injury, imagine that it's being used more and more to do "facelifts" for the very wealthy, because not only can it lower blood pressure and get rid of migraines, it can diminish wrinkles, too. And so what ought to be an inexpensive treasure for everyone, especially in dire economic times, has become an overpriced luxury for a very few. Doesn't it sound like it might be time to talk about a revolution?

Congratulations, you've just imagined the community acupuncture movement!

We are writing this book because we started the revolution, put the community acupuncture movement in motion, and we believe that it could go so much farther than it has already. Acupuncture is not only valuable because it is an extremely inexpensive, nonpharmaceutical therapy for pain and stress, but because it challenges the way we think about healthcare. Its profound simplicity is an antidote for the greed and bureaucracy that have created the American healthcare crisis. Community acupuncture is, by its very nature, healthcare reform. This is why so many people are so excited about it.

There are a lot of books about acupuncture, but none of them are as simple as this one. Our critics will undoubtedly be horrified at what they consider our oversimplification of acupuncture. However, the contributors to this book have more than forty years of collective experience doing acupuncture, and all of us have been treating more than fifty patients every week for years now. We do a lot of acupuncture; it's how we make our living. When you do something with intense focus for a long time, you are able to see it with clarity, and what originally seemed complex and overwhelming becomes simple and transparent. It is this simplicity and transparency we want to share particularly with patients and new acupuncturists.

We also believe that there is a great need to create a different culture around the practice of acupuncture. Instead of acupuncture being esoteric and inaccessible, it could be widely embraced and appreciated. Part of what can create that embrace and appreciation is understanding, and so we want you to feel that you share in the understanding we have acquired over years of practice. We want you to feel that you understand some basic and essential truths about acupuncture: what it is, how it works, why people need it. Instead of acupuncture being some kind of overpriced, exotic, New Age indulgence, it could be humble, universal, and infinitely useful. We hope that this book provides the recipe for that transformation.

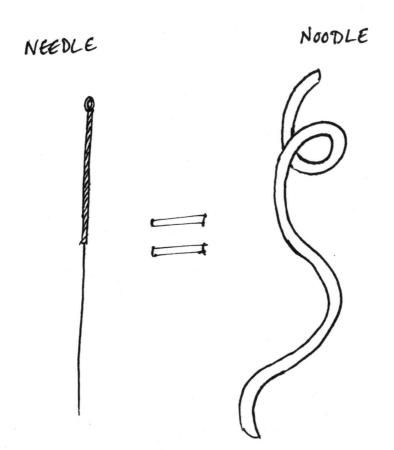

Part One: Acupuncture is Like Noodles

Part One: Acupuncture is Like Noodles

Acupuncture is the practice of inserting tiny needles under the skin at specific points in order to stimulate the body's ability to heal itself. The most important thing about acupuncture is not why it works, but how amazingly well it works.

Acupuncture is effective for an enormously wide range of conditions, so wide that it is likely that it will help almost any problem to some degree, even if it can't cure it entirely. For instance, in our experience, acupuncture can: decrease inflammation, calm spasms, boost immunity, increase fertility, induce labor, dispel a migraine, shrink swelling, relieve pain in almost any location, regulate hormones, cut recovery time from surgery almost in half, calm anxiety, lift depression, restore mobility, improve digestion, and create deep relaxation. That's only a partial list.

Besides being effective for a lot of different specific conditions, acupuncture is beneficial in some general ways for everyone: it usually improves sleep, energy, and mood, as well as reducing stress.

People often think about acupuncture as being effective for complex, difficult, relatively uncommon problems that Western medicine has limited success with, such as AIDS, multiple sclerosis, or the aftereffects of a stroke. In reality, though, acupuncture is just as suited to treating garden-variety problems like headaches, indigestion, and PMS. The reason that acupuncture is sometimes effective for complex and unusual conditions is that it is basically somewhat effective for everything, not because acupuncture itself is complex and unusual.

Acupuncture is particularly helpful for people with chronic diseases, meaning conditions that can be managed but not cured. Because these people often need to take many medications with multiple side effects, acupuncture can greatly improve their quality of life by helping them with their mood, their energy, and their sleep – without creating any more side effects.

Acupuncture is a very safe form of medicine. Because it depends on the body's ability to heal itself, acupuncture cannot make a problem worse. Acupuncture is very gentle in that way; usually it helps a lot, but in the unlikely event that it doesn't help, it can't hurt, either.

Acupuncture is so ancient that nobody knows for sure where or how it originated. Acupuncture is not necessarily Chinese or even Asian in origin. Acupuncture does not fit well into any Western medical paradigm. Acupuncture has been practiced for so long in so many places that there are an almost infinite variety of ways to do it. Many of those different ways are based on mutually contradictory concepts, but they all work. They all reduce pain and stress, and they all improve sleep, energy, and mood.

Just as nobody knows where acupuncture originated, nobody really knows why it works.

There are many theories about acupuncture. The ancient Chinese, while they may not have invented acupuncture, developed an elaborate theoretical foundation for it. More recently, Western medical research has suggested biomedical mechanisms for acupuncture. None of these theories, no matter how interesting they are, actually explain why inserting tiny needles under the skin stimulates the body's ability to heal itself. None of the theories explain how they can all contradict each other, and yet all of them still work.

Acupuncture is not like any other form of "alternative medicine". It is unique. It is nothing like chiropractic treatment, or massage therapy, or naturopathic medicine. It is not like Western medical interventions such as surgery or physical therapy. It should not be compared or confused with any of these things.

Acupuncture is somewhat like prayer, in that sometimes you get a lot more than you asked for, in ways that you never expected, through the action of forces that you can't see.

Acupuncture is also somewhat like food. Providing acupuncture is like cooking and receiving acupuncture is like eating. The ingredients are all contained within the body itself; the acupuncture treatment is a way of arranging them so that the body can use them better. Once the acupuncturist arranges the needles in the right combinations, the patient's job is to sit quietly long enough to "digest" the treatment.

Acupuncture nourishes the body by helping it to relax.

Besides being like food in general, acupuncture is a lot like noodles, in particular. The oldest written accounts of noodles come from ancient China, but the Chinese did not necessarily invent noodles. Noodles are made from many different ingredients, all over the world, and prepared in widely different ways. Noodles and acupuncture are both flexible, nourishing, and potentially very, very inexpensive.

About Acupuncture in America

Acupuncture probably first came to America with Chinese immigrant laborers. Acupuncture began to "become mainstream", which really means "become interesting to white people" after Nixon's trip to China.

In the 1980s it began to be possible to go to school and get a degree to become an acupuncturist, instead of becoming an acupuncturist by apprenticing in a clinic. This is not unlike going to chef school to get a degree in culinary arts, versus learning to make noodles by helping your grandmother in the kitchen.

Soon after this, it became possible to take out student loans to go to acupuncture school, and after that, the price of acupuncture education went through the roof. Many students now graduate from acupuncture school with $100,000 or more in debt. This is not unlike culinary students, who graduate from chef school burdened with huge student loans, when all they really wanted to do was to learn how to cook.

Unlike chefs, there are virtually no jobs for acupuncturists. This is partly a result of most Americans, including acupuncturists and acupuncture schools, not understanding how acupuncture is like noodles. Like noodles, acupuncture is most useful in the plural, not the singular.

Although we do not know why acupuncture works, we do know a few things about how it works best. Acupuncture usually requires a series of treatments to work. For acute problems, such as a sprained ankle, it's a short series of treatments; for chronic problems, such as migraine headaches, it's a long series, possibly requiring months of treatments. For severe, chronic problems such as autoimmune diseases, acupuncture is effective but might require regular, ongoing treatment for years or decades.

If acupuncture is like food, then a problem is like hunger, the body needing something. If it is a small, recent hunger such as a sprained ankle, a small amount of food will do the trick. If it is a deep, old, long-standing hunger, then the problem demands regular doses of nourishment as often as possible.

A big reason that there are almost no jobs for acupuncturists is that, once acupuncture became interesting to white people, it began to be priced in a very unfortunate way. Although acupuncture requires frequent, regular repetition to be effective, most acupuncture treatments cost $65 to $150. Since a single treatment costs this much, a series of ten treatments costs $650 to $1500. Since almost no one can afford this, almost no one in America gets acupuncture.

This is like almost no one getting fed, when almost everyone is hungry. Almost everyone suffers from stress in some way, and almost everyone could be helped by acupuncture.

Some patients who try acupuncture stop after one or two treatments because they can't afford to continue and they aren't getting good results. This is like eating only a single noodle for lunch when what you need is a bowl of spaghetti, or like taking only two pills out of a prescribed ten-day series of antibiotics. Of course there won't be any good results.

What good to anyone is a single, overpriced noodle?

Since acupuncturists know how to give people something that they need, we believe that this means they have an obligation to do so. The knowledge of how to do acupuncture cannot be separated from a responsibility to use it unselfishly.

The great 6th century Chinese acupuncturist Sun Simiao, who was known as "the King of Medicine", wrote:

> Whenever a great physician treats diseases, he has to be mentally calm and his disposition firm. He should not give way to wishes and desires, but has to develop first a marked attitude of compassion. He should commit himself firmly to the willingness to take the effort to save every living creature. If someone seeks help because of illness, or on the ground of another difficulty, a great physician should not pay attention to status, wealth, or age; neither should he question whether the particular person is attractive or unattractive, whether he is an enemy or a friend, whether he is Chinese or a foreigner, or finally, whether he

is uneducated or educated. He should meet everyone on equal ground; he should always act as if he were thinking of himself. He should not desire anything and should ignore all consequences; he is not to ponder over his own fortune or misfortune and thus preserve life and have compassion for it. He should look upon those who have come to grief as if he himself had been struck, and he should sympathize with them deep in his heart.[1]

Acupuncture cannot be understood correctly apart from the moral and social responsibilities that accompany it, but in America, these moral and social responsibilities are widely ignored. It's time to ask: what would Sun Simiao do?

The Social Responsibility of Noodles

Here is a letter that we recently received from a patient:

To Whom it May Concern,

I started coming to Working Class Acupuncture for treatment about a month and a half ago. I had experienced a severe manic episode in June of this year, and had also been assaulted on (public transit) during this time period. Due to (this) incident, my left arm had lost functionality, and would hang limp by my side when it was overexerted doing regular activities. Alternating heat and ice and exercising/stretching it did nothing. I lost my job due to the manic episode, and was left with no health insurance. Fearing that my arm would be partially paralyzed, I scrambled to locate a physician or chiropractor that could assist, but on my unemployment income, help was not available. Acting on a recommendation, I began coming to WCA.

To my surprise, I noticed a slight difference almost immediately. Continual weekly treatments by Skip have restored functioning to my left arm, and the pain has almost disappeared. I was surprised to catch myself holding a bag full of groceries in my left arm the other day - something I had not been able to do for months. I can also steer my car with both hands now. The improvement - actually, the restoration of mobility in my left arm to pre-accident state - has truly been a miracle. I was really afraid that I would not be able to use my arm well again.

Along with the above issues, I also suffer from scoliosis and fibromyalgia. Acupuncture has seriously aided in my ability to comfortably move and function, and lessened the amount of pain experienced on a regular basis. The main health issue that is occurring at this time for me is depression, which is an expected biochemical downswing from the mania I suffered this summer. Although on medication for the disorder, the depression has been debilitating. Acupuncture treatments have aided tremendously with this serious issue as well.

I am so grateful to Skip for his expert assistance. WCA has really helped me to get it together, and has given me hope. The peaceful and serene atmosphere; the kindness and professionalism of all who work there, and the awesome effectiveness of acupuncture treatment is really mind-boggling. I feel so, so fortunate. I'm incredibly appreciative that this healing - which is so priceless - has been made available to me on my really limited income. I don't really know how to adequately express my thanks for the recovery, treatment and support I've received from WCA, and have hopes that with continual treatment I will have fewer issues with bi-polar disorder and fibromyalgia in the future. I am forever indebted. Please express my sincere gratitude to Skip, along with the rest of the fantastic folks at WCA. See you Saturday!

Many, many people are suffering from stress, injuries, or emotional problems that make it difficult for them to work. If acupuncture can help people recover and return to work, acupuncturists have a social responsibility to help them, particularly at a time of economic difficulty for the entire country. In some cases, acupuncture can have even more dramatic effects, as another of our patients writes:

My husband was diagnosed with metastatic lung cancer in 1993. He had surgery and radiation, and responded pretty well, but by 1999 he was on hospice. We were introduced to acupuncture because at that time Kaiser Hospice offered five in-home acupuncture treatments to patient and caregiver. I wanted to try it, but my husband was reluctant. He did it for me, because I couldn't get it unless he got it too. Once he tried it, he liked it very much. He was looking for anything positive he could find, to help him keep fighting, and it made him feel better. We looked forward to the acupuncturist coming every week.

When the five treatments were up, he wanted to keep getting acupuncture, and the hospice nurses found a facility that would continue the treatments on a sliding-fee scale. Otherwise we could never have afforded it; we were on OHP and Medicare. He wanted to reduce the amount of morphine he was taking, partly because the Medicare laws had changed and it had gotten really expensive for us.

We got acupuncture once a week for three years, and then twice a week for two more years. As a result of getting acupuncture once a week, he got off Oxycodone completely, and reduced his total narcotic use by 70%. He gradually got better; he started mowing the lawn, trimming the hedges, playing golf. We traveled, and he didn't get a wheelchair at the airport, he would walk. He gradually came back to living a fairly normal life. He would get winded, of course. But he went fishing. He babysat our grandson. We would leave acupuncture and go do errands all day. His health would always get worse in the winter, but acupuncture would pull him through.
Each time he got a treatment, it would give him the energy to go until the next treatment. It sustained him. It calmed him. It gave him the will to continue to fight.

It added five years to his life.

When we started getting acupuncture twice a week, his energy really progressed, and he started doing something he hadn't done in a long time, which was playing music. He was a drummer. He played with some famous jazz musicians when he was younger. He loved to play. Music was a big part of his life. It was so good for him. I can't tell you how much enjoyment he got out of it. He would say that when he played, he felt 17 and not 70.

He always used visualization, and he prayed constantly. Acupuncture worked along with all of the faith that he had. Acupuncture was a piece of the puzzle that made up the whole picture -- along with prayer and visualization and music -- the whole picture of five more years of living together, of being happy, and without acupuncture, that picture would not have been there.

As far as being the caregiver, acupuncture gave me a calmness -- not just because of the treatments themselves, but in knowing that my husband was doing something for himself. It was something we shared together. I'm going to keep doing acupuncture because it gives me energy and I know it's preventing bigger health problems. I don't want to take pills for every little thing. I want to be able to control my own health with any alternative that's reasonable to me.

Just as there are many different ways to cook a meal, there are many different ways to practice acupuncture. No one way can be called right while another way is called wrong. Very few people would think that it makes any sense to say that some Japanese udon noodle soup is "right" while Italian minestrone noodle soup is "wrong". Individuals might have preferences, but any style of cooking can be delicious and nourishing. And a hungry person will be most concerned that he can get enough noodles to eat.

If noodles could add five years to someone's life, or give someone back his ability to work, and you had the ability to make noodles, wouldn't you think you also had an obligation to make noodles? And wouldn't you also think that you had an obligation to make noodles in such as way that they were affordable to as many people as possible?

Of course, you could make very elaborate, expensive noodle creations and serve them in five-star restaurants where only rich people could afford to eat, which would mean that only a few people got any noodles. Or you could come up with recipes for noodles that use simple ingredients, and serve them in unpretentious settings, so that as many people as possible could afford to eat noodles. It would be your choice, but there are social and moral implications to what you do with your noodles.

Making Simple Noodles: the Kitchen and the Dining Room

At Working Class Acupuncture, we developed what is now called "the community acupuncture business model". This basically means that we figured out how to make inexpensive, simple noodles and provide them to a lot of people. Of course, we then began to encourage any other acupuncturist who would listen to us to do the same thing. This is how the revolution got started.

Many other acupuncturists were interested in simple noodles, and so after a while we helped create what is now called the Community Acupuncture Network, a nonprofit organization to support acupuncturists who are using the community acupuncture business model. CAN has a website, www.communityacupuncturenetwork.org, and patients looking for affordable acupuncture can find a list of clinics there, while acupuncturists looking for help can find more information about the community acupuncture business model.

There are two different stages to making simple noodles: how to prepare them and how to serve them, or what you do in the kitchen and what you do in the dining room. What you do in the kitchen is equivalent to the way you use acupuncture clinically: how you diagnose problems, how you decide where to put the needles, every aspect of treating a patient with acupuncture. What you do in the dining room is equivalent to how you set up your business: what you charge, what your clinic looks like, every aspect of running a business. This book will describe the most important aspects of what we do in our kitchen and what we do in our dining room. Of course, all of this originates with social and moral concerns about how to provide noodles to as many people as possible. You can't understand what we do without understanding why we want to do it.

> As acupuncturists, we control who has access to our services and we communicate this by where we set up our practices, the environments we create in our offices, the clothes we wear to work, the language we use to talk about what we do, the fees we charge, and how we envision the future of our medicine.
> -- Cris Monteiro, Providence Community Acupuncture

Class and Noodles

We believe that being socially responsible acupuncturists requires us to specifically address issues of socioeconomic class. Which, in America, is not easy to do, since class in America is often invisible, hard to pin down, and uncomfortable for people to talk about. However, most sociologists agree that class is a reality in America, and many also agree about the basic class structure:

> Upper class/Ruling class/Owning class
> Upper Middle Class
> Middle Class
> Lower Middle Class
> Working Class
> Underclass/Low Income/Chronic Poverty[2]

Defining these classes precisely is much more challenging. A majority of Americans, when asked, will define themselves as "middle class". Census figures, however, tell a much different story. According to a recent survey on the U.S. Census website[3], four-fifths of U.S. households earn less than $100,000 per year (gross, not net). Since a household is defined as roughly three people, and a comfortable, truly middle class lifestyle is hard to imagine for three people with less than a gross income of $100,000 a year (considering the cost of health insurance alone), this suggests that four-fifths of U.S. households are actually lower middle class, working class, or underclass.

Classism is defined as bias based on socioeconomic status. In a nutshell, classism is a set of beliefs that define people as superior or inferior depending on their social position, wealth, education, and culture. Classism may be internalized, meaning that a working class person may believe herself to be inherently less worthy than an upper middle class person. Classism may be subtle and systematic, resulting in working class people and their concerns being invisible, or noticeable mostly by their absence.

Values differ across classes, in part because the structure of people's lives varies enormously based on their resources.[4] While some values are common to all classes -- everyone values friendship and social connection, for instance -- how those values are expressed may differ as well. An extension of classism is the belief that the values held by the upper class and the upper middle class are the "right" or "correct" values, and the way those classes do things represent the "best" way to do things. This is yet another way of making lower middle class, working class, and low income people invisible.

Since classism is hard to talk about, over the years we have developed some strategies. We have been especially interested in finding ways to articulate how values differ across classes, since those values inform how we provide acupuncture. Those values shape how we operate both in the kitchen, the clinical aspect of our acupuncture practice, and the dining room, the business aspect of our acupuncture practice. One of our strategies to articulate different values across classes is an imaginative exercise which we will call "Party Noodles".[5]

People of all classes value socializing, and people of all classes go to parties. Also, people of all classes eat noodles. To do this exercise, you will have to imagine a woman of each social class getting ready to go to a party at which noodles will be served. How she gets ready, what the party is like, and what kind of noodles are there will help you identify the values which are important to her class. A note: all of the values that we focus on in this exercise are positive, since the point of the exercise is not to prove that any class is better than any other, just that values differ.

So, imagine a woman from the upper/ruling/owning class getting ready for a party. What kind of party is it? Perhaps a gala to raise funds for a new wing at the hospital, held at an art museum or at someone's country estate. How did she receive her invitation? Her personal assistant or social secretary gave it to her, and someone else's social secretary sent it. How did she get on the guest list? Because of who she is. What will she wear? A dress that was probably designed for her, which she will never wear again. Did she pay for the dress? Unlikely; probably a designer gave it to her, just in hopes that she would be photographed wearing it. Who made the noodles at the party? Someone's personal chef, from a recipe invented for the occasion, possibly including truffles. The upper class values that this experience reflects: *elegance, status, personal service, refinement, individuality, beauty, exoticism, uniqueness*. Limitations on resources? Virtually none.

Now imagine a woman from the upper middle class getting ready for a party. She is, say, a psychiatrist. What kind of party is it? Maybe a cocktail party at a country club. How did she receive her invitation? In the mail, on expensive stationery. How did she get on the guest list? Through her professional connections. What will she wear? A suit bought for the occasion with a recognizable designer label. Will she wear it again? Yes, at a similar occasion, at a decent interval in the future. Who made the noodles at the party? The chef at the country club, from a classic recipe. The upper middle class values that this experience reflects: *professionalism, status, personal achievement, conformity, respectability, tastefulness*. Limitations on resources? Few.

The "middle-middle class" is so hard to define, so mixed in with the upper-middle class on one end and the lower-middle class on the other, that for the purposes of this exercise we just skip it, and go on to imagine a lower middle class woman, say the psychiatrist's office manager, getting ready for a party. What kind of party is it? Perhaps a baby shower at a family friend's house. How did she receive her invitation? By email. How did she get on the guest list? Her family relationships. What will she wear? A dress that she chose originally for its durability and value, which she has worn before and will wear again. Who made the noodles at the party? Her sister, who is throwing the party for a friend, using a family recipe that she knows everyone likes. The lower middle class values that this experience reflects: *family connections, frugality, hard work, stability, simplicity, ease*. Limitations on resources? Significant.

How about a working class woman getting ready for a party? A night shift cleaner in the hospital for which the upper class woman is raising money. What kind of party is it? A birthday party for a friend. How did she receive her invitation? Her friend asked her. How did she get on the guest list? She and her friends always do things like this together; there was no guest list. What will she wear? A dress that she made herself, or found in a thrift store, or borrowed from another friend. Who made the noodles at the party? Everyone; it's a potluck. The working class values that this experience reflects: *interdependence, creativity, hard work, resourcefulness, personal relationships, directness, loyalty.* Limitations on resources? Enormous.

Like the middle-middle class, the underclass is hard to define in terms of values because it is fragmented and hard to define, period. The community acupuncture business model as we have designed it does not, unfortunately, make acupuncture accessible to underclass people, since it depends on a stable, consistent patient base and a fee for service structure. Our understanding of the underclass is that it is defined by a lack of stability. Chronic poverty is a chaotic experience. It is unlikely that someone who is not able to have a stable living situation, someone who is continually dealing with crises, would be able to commit to regularly paying for acupuncture. In Portland, there are a number of non-profit clinics that provide acupuncture to underclass people, some of them through existing public health programs. The challenges of providing consistent, quality acupuncture treatment to underclass people are significantly different from the challenges of providing the same thing to working class people. We believe that we have been successful in figuring out how to offer acupuncture to working class people because we come from working class backgrounds ourselves; the most qualified person to design a model to offer acupuncture to underclass people would be an activist from an underclass background. (Of course, the sheer cost of acupuncture education is a significant limitation in terms of who enters the profession in the first place.) We wish that we were able to address the challenges of providing acupuncture to underclass people in this book and this business model, but we aren't; the best we can do for underclass patients at this point is to offer referrals to other programs.

Two Types of Noodles

Once you are at least willing to entertain the idea that people of different classes might value different things, it's time to think about what kind of values conventional acupuncture practices reflect. For an industry such as acupuncture (although it is a very small industry indeed), it is easiest to see its values by looking at its marketing. If conventional acupuncture is also a noodle, it is marketed in two distinct varieties: the Zen-Spa Noodle, and the White-Coat Noodle. These noodles reflect, respectively, the "alternative" and the "complementary" aspects of acupuncture, and combined they define acupuncture as "complementary and alternative medicine".

The Zen-Spa Noodle, or the Alternative Noodle, is a delicate noodle embossed with gold-leaf Chinese characters. The Zen-Spa Noodle is acupuncture marketed as an exotic spa service for the discerning consumer. The Zen-Spa Noodle reaches its apex with "facial rejuvenation acupuncture", otherwise known as "the acupuncture facelift", otherwise known as "acupuncture for people who have nothing really wrong with them but want to spend a lot of money anyway". Marketing for the Zen-Spa Noodle features elegant, softly lit treatment rooms, descriptions of personalized treatments, lots of one-on-one attention from an acupuncturist, exquisite Asian-esque images of Buddhas, fountains and bamboo, altogether evoking the idea of a special therapy for special people. Let's see: *elegance, status, personal service, refinement, individuality, beauty, exoticism, uniqueness.* Who is the Zen-Spa Noodle for? One hint: it's not for the night cleaner at the hospital.

The White-Coat Noodle, on the other hand, is a noodle sturdy enough to be wrapped up in the red tape of medical bureaucracy. The White-Coat Noodle is acupuncture marketed as complementary medicine, nothing weird or scary, nice and safe with reassuring pictures of serious acupuncturists in lab coats wearing stethoscopes. (There is absolutely no reason on earth an acupuncturist would need a stethoscope.) Other marketing props besides stethoscopes are as many letters behind the acupuncturist's name as possible, a tastefully furnished but suitably sterile office, research studies showing the effectiveness and respectability of acupuncture, and insurance billing just like you have at your M.D.'s office. The acupuncturist may even demonstrate further expertise by "specializing" in women's health, or sports medicine, or pain management. Hmm, what's that? *Professionalism, status, personal achievement, conformity, respectability, tastefulness. . .* one guess as to who the White-Coat Noodle is for? And no, it's not the night cleaner at the hospital, and not the office manager either.

The Zen-Spa Noodle is acupuncture designed for the upper class, reflecting upper class values, and the White-Coat Noodle is acupuncture designed for the upper middle class, reflecting upper middle class values. The price tags attached to the Zen-Spa Noodle and the White-Coat Noodle confirm that their target markets are the wealthy. Since conventional acupuncture marketing presents only the Zen-Spa Noodle and the White-Coat Noodle as acceptable ways of doing acupuncture, apparently there are no noodles for the night cleaner at the hospital and the office manager.

When challenged about this lack of noodles, conventional acupuncturists often offer reprehensible suggestions that working class and lower middle class people do not really "value their health"; if they did, they would be willing to forego necessities like electricity and groceries in order to spend $100 or so to buy a single noodle, either a lovely gold-embossed noodle or a noodle respectably wrapped in red tape. This is a good example of classism in action. $100 represents a much greater portion of a working class or lower middle class person's resources than that of an upper middle class or upper class person. If you earn $25,000 a year, $100 represents about 7% of your monthly take home pay. 7% of the take home pay for someone who earns $150,000 a year is about $600. Would the psychiatrist be accused of not valuing her health if she had qualms about paying $600 for a single acupuncture treatment? Even this comparison fails to take into account the greater proportion of a working class person's wages that must go to basic living expenses, relative to an upper middle class person's. The psychiatrist probably could pay $600 for an acupuncture treatment on a regular basis without getting her electricity shut off or having to eat less; the night cleaner at the hospital would not be so lucky if she tried to regularly get acupuncture at $100 per treatment. And yet it is somehow the night cleaner's *fault* that she is not getting acupuncture; her values are the problem. Because when it comes to values, the psychiatrist's values are somehow better, more correct, and more real than the night cleaner's.

Acupuncturists: Use Your Noodles!

If you are an acupuncturist reading this book, we hope it is occurring to you that what people value is inextricably connected to the resources they have. We also hope that you are thinking that it makes no sense at all from a business perspective to position acupuncture so that it is accessible and appealing only to that one-fifth of the population with almost unlimited resources. It's not only morally questionable, it's plain dumb, because that one-fifth is much too small a market. If you want to make acupuncture genuinely accessible to the other four-fifths of the population, however, one thing you must do is to think hard about what acupuncture would look like if it were designed around lower middle class and working class values. Working class people and lower middle class people do not use acupuncture primarily because they can't afford it, but even if they could afford the Zen-Spa Noodle and the White-Coat Noodle, they might find those noodles uncomfortable and off-putting. Can you get the Zen-Spa Noodle and the White-Coat Noodle out of your thoughts enough to imagine another kind of Noodle, an Unpretentious Noodle, a Humble and

Delicious Noodle, a Noodle based on values like: *family connections, frugality, hard work, stability, simplicity, ease, interdependence, creativity, resourcefulness, personal relationships, directness, and loyalty?*

Try, OK? Because that is the point of the rest of this book.

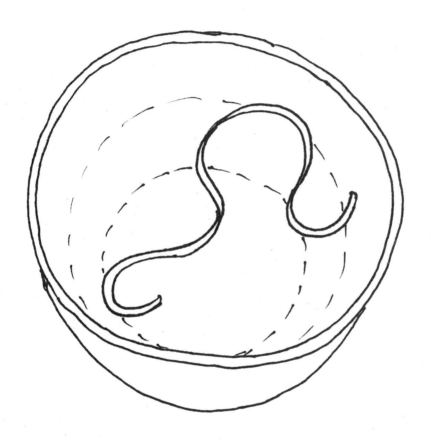

Part Two: Welcome to Our Kitchen

Before we give you a tour of the kitchen in which we strive to produce our Humble and Delicious Noodles, we need to clarify some of our basic principles. As we said earlier: acupuncture is like food. Providing acupuncture is like cooking and receiving acupuncture is like eating. The ingredients are all contained within the body itself; the acupuncture treatment is a way of arranging them so that the body can use them better. Once the acupuncturist arranges the needles in the right combinations, the patient's job is to sit quietly long enough to "digest" the treatment. To understand how we think about the clinical aspect of providing acupuncture, it's most important to understand that the acupuncturist is not adding or subtracting anything to or from the patient's body.

In the Chinese theories of acupuncture, one of the most fundamental concepts is that of "qi", pronounced "chee". There is no one equivalent word or phrase for qi in English. This is very unfortunate, because one of the best ways to describe what acupuncture does is to say that it moves qi.

The Chinese character for qi originated with three horizontal brushstrokes, representing water vapor rising to form clouds, so qi originally meant something like mist, something not quite solid, something moving. Over time the character evolved to include the image of steam rising from rice, specifically rice cooked for guests, and so the concept of qi came to include the idea of giving, and the idea of nourishment.[1] Weather in China is sometimes described as "the big qi", while soda pop is "qi water". Qi cannot be located, but it can be felt; it's fizz, and like the weather, it's all around. Qi can also be translated as breath, atmosphere, function, knowing-how, and connectivity.[2]

When acupuncturists put needles in, they are usually trying to "get qi". On a very basic level, this means that the patient feels something where the needles are, something distinct from pain, *something happening*. The sensation can be described as fullness, pressure, tingling, or a dull ache. (Needles do not need to go in deeply in order to get qi. Many acupuncturists at our clinic get qi by inserting needles only a few millimeters under the skin.) One patient, having his first-ever acupuncture treatment, described it as "a warm hum." We believe that getting qi means increasing circulation in the body, circulation not only of tangible substances like blood but of intangible non-substances such as awareness, information, intention, and strength.

One of the effects of acupuncture should be to get all the different parts of the patient communicating. We should explain a little more what we mean by that, which requires a bit of discussion of what Americans like to call "the mind-body connection". Anyone who practices acupuncture for a while will notice that one of its unusual effects is apparently to make connections between the conscious and the unconscious mind. Patients commonly report having sudden insights about their problems while getting acupuncture: shifts in understanding, vivid intuitions about what they need to do, clear communication from what some call "the Inner Physician". Exactly how putting tiny little needles under the skin accomplishes all that is something that naturally we would all love to know, and of course nobody has the slightest idea. Sometimes people explain it by invoking "the mind-body connection". Interestingly enough, though, that whole concept makes no sense in a universe that includes qi. There can be no mind-body connection, because there was never any separation in the first place. A human being is a continuum, with one end being dense and physical, the other end being ethereal and spiritual. Both ends depend on qi to animate them, and qi is also everything in the middle of the continuum that is not quite physical and not quite spiritual. Qi is the warm hum of being alive.

As we noted earlier, acupuncture is not like other forms of medicine. It is particularly not like other forms of Chinese medicine like herbology, which requires intricate knowledge of the yin and yang qualities of herbs and how to balance those qualities in a formula. Patients sometimes state their reason for coming in to the clinic as being in need of "balancing", and these patients tend to believe that what we acupuncturists are trying to do with the needles is to balance their energy. (Qi is sometimes mistranslated as "energy".) What we are actually trying to do is much simpler than that, however: mostly we are just trying to get things moving all along the continuum. Qi means knowing-how; getting qi means helping the body remember to do what it knows how to do. There's no need to tell it, to manipulate it, or to force it.

To an acupuncturist, all forms of pain or illness mean that things have somehow gotten stuck: somehow, qi is just not moving. The essence of acupuncture diagnosis, as we understand it (and remember, acupuncture diagnosis and Chinese herbal diagnosis are not the same at all) is in identifying what is most stuck; if what is most stuck can become freer, everything else along the continuum that is a human being will become freer too. It's like dominoes -- to introduce yet another metaphor. Acupuncture diagnosis is all about identifying that first domino, so that you can tip it over with your needles. Here's the thing, though: all kinds of acupuncture diagnosis work. There is no one right way to identify that first domino. Any domino that you tip over is going to tip over another one, and any domino that tips over is going to result in a person feeling better.

All human problems share an element of stagnation. Stagnation creates tension; tension also creates stagnation. When acupuncture gets things moving, people usually relax. Being relaxed, in turn, is replenishing. An acupuncturist does not need to try to micromanage the specifics of how the body balances, regulates, and heals itself; just getting things moving again is always a big step in the right direction. It really is that simple.

Thank You, Michael Pollan

On January 28, 2007, an article by Michael Pollan appeared in the New York Times, titled "Unhappy Meals". It began with the suggestion that the supposedly impossibly difficult question of how people should eat healthfully could be simplifed to three basic instructions: eat food (as opposed to non-food), in reasonable quantities, mostly the kind that originates in the vegetable as opposed to the animal kingdom. We promptly printed out multiple copies of the article and flung them around our waiting room, in hopes that our patients would read these wise words. We love the article "Unhappy Meals" most, however, not for its practical advice about healthy eating, but for the way it adds depth and dimension to our acupuncture-as-food metaphor. Everything that Pollan writes concerning our confusion about how to eat is true, ten times over, for our confusion about how to use acupuncture. We have misunderstood acupuncture in the very same ways that we have misunderstood food.

If you haven't read the article, we encourage you to do so; you can search for it on the New York Times website. Briefly, though, Pollan's arguments go something like this: about twenty years ago, instead of talking about food in terms of food, people began talking about food in terms of nutrients, as if the most important thing about any food must be the nutrients that it contains. This was a positive development for nutritional scientists and big food companies who use the idea of nutrients in their marketing, but not so positive for the rest of us who eat food as opposed to nutrients. While nutrients can be broken down and isolated in a laboratory, foods can't; foods often behave in the human body very differently than the nutrients that they contain. For example, researchers theorized that the reason that a diet rich in fruits and vegetables seems to protect people against cancer is because fruits and vegetables contain antioxidants. Enterprising supplement companies promptly began manufacturing antioxidant supplements and marketing them as cancer preventatives. Unfortunately, however, it turns out that once you take the antioxidants out of the foods, they have different effects: for example, taking beta carotene supplements seems to actually increase people's risk for certain cancers.

Even the simplest food is extraordinarily complex, full of many different chemical compounds that are constantly changing. Reductionist science, applied to food, means trying to break food down into its component parts and then study those parts one at a time. The problem here is that this requires ignoring all of the relationships amongst those parts, as well as the reality that a food might be not only more than, but completely different from, the sum of its chemical, "nutrient" parts. Which means that understanding nutrients is not the key to understanding food. Any food is an almost infinitely complex whole, which interacts with the human body as another almost infinitely complex whole.

Just because we can isolate and study nutrients does not mean that we have food and what it does in the body all figured out. When science first identified carbohydrates, proteins and fats, people thought they knew almost everything that there was to know about food; then science identified vitamins a few decades later, and everyone thought vitamins were the key; now it's polyphenols and carotenoids that have center stage in the scientific dramatic mystery of food. But, Pollan writes, how can we fathom the inner heart of even such a basic food as, say, a carrot? Fortunately, the person eating the carrot doesn't need to, which is what defines the difference between eating food and eating nutrients. You do not need to understand the carrot's intricacies in order to benefit from eating it. You just need to eat it.[3]

Isn't that beautiful? You don't need to penetrate the mysteries of something mysterious in order to use it! And in the case of acupuncture, whose impenetrable mechanisms combined with its ancient origins make it potentially unfathomable altogether, the attempts to apply reductive science to its workings have created actual obstacles to people reaping its benefits. *You can't break down acupuncture in order to understand it – and you really can't break down acupuncture if you have any intention of using it to do any good for the people who need it the most.*

People do try, unfortunately. On the one hand, there are the materialists, people who believe that if we can't quantify something, it isn't there. These are the people who react to the idea of qi with apoplectic rage, who rail about superstition, who think acupuncture should have a "scientific basis" before anyone is allowed to use it. We tend to believe, as in the case of food, establishing a "scientific basis" for acupuncture may not do anyone any particular good, except the scientists who get the research grants.

And on the other hand, we have the acupuncturists who react to the ranting materialists with their own attempts to fathom acupuncture's complexity. They retort that acupuncture is indeed founded on science, just not the Western, double-blind research variety. They justify acupuncture based on its roots in Chinese culture and philosophy; they demand that anyone who practices acupuncture do so on the basis of thousands of hours studying Chinese medical theories. They treat the concept of qi with near-religious reverence.

We think all of them are missing the point. We don't want to attack the idea of qi, nor do we want to defend it. We don't care much about the idea of qi at all – we just want to use qi itself, for the people who need it. It's not that we have any doubts about the intrinsic worth of scientific research or of the study of Chinese philosophy. It's just that neither of those things necessarily has anything to do with the practice of acupuncture. We are about to try to explain how we use acupuncture clinically. We want to make it clear that using acupuncture clinically, and doing it well, so that people get better, has nothing to do with taking the components of acupuncture apart to see how they tick -- whether those are biochemical components or Chinese philosophical components, it makes no difference to the patient how they tick. Food may contain nutrients, but nutrients are not the reason that we need food. Acupuncture may release endorphins or raise the yang, but those are not reasons to receive acupuncture. Like food, acupuncture is infinitely more than the sum of its parts. We know how to arrange certain parts so that good things result, but we can't analyze the parts or even the results, and we think it's basically a mistake to try.

Acupuncture, like a carrot, functions perfectly well as a whole, unfathomed mystery. And just as growing a carrot and chopping it up in a salad requires infinitely fewer resources than manufacturing a beta-carotene supplement, there are ways to provide acupuncture that can make it available to people of limited resources. These ways also tend to leave acupuncture intact, by simply using it as if it were whole in itself rather than breaking it down into component parts and trying to manipulate those parts. Analysis of something unfathomable is expensive, time consuming, and a highly questionable priority when people are hungry. One of our choices as acupuncturists is to stop talking, stop thinking, stop analyzing and *just shut up and feed people.*

Ingredients and Recipes

It isn't difficult to feed people. To continue with our clinic as kitchen metaphor, the ingredients that we use are the acupuncture points on the body. In Traditional Chinese Medicine, there are some 500 recognized acupuncture points. (What exactly is an acupuncture point? The place where you insert an acupuncture needle. Really, that is about as precise a definition as you can hope to get. We know *where* they are, but we don't know exactly *what* they are.[4]) Since there are many other systems of acupuncture besides Traditional Chinese Medicine, there are probably thousands of other points according to those other systems. (This might be one reason why some research studies show that "placebo acupuncture" is just as effective as any other kind, and more effective than drugs: who's to say that the "non-acupuncture points" chosen by scientists for the control group are not real acupuncture points according to some unknown tradition?)

In our efforts to make what we do simple and inexpensive, there is no possibility that we could use all or even most of the acupuncture points that we know. Furthermore, there is no need to do so. Just as you can make a wonderful meal out of a few simple ingredients -- say, spaghetti with olive oil, sauteed garlic, and some coarse black pepper -- you can create a wonderful acupuncture treatment by using a few simple points. Like most home cooking, our acupuncture relies on using some of the same basic ingredients in different combinations. A tour of our kitchen includes a list of our favorite ingredients, along with our favorite recipes.

But First: Thank You, NADA

For the most exquisitely simple noodles of all, and the best example of how easy it is to feed people with acupuncture, if you are really serious about it.

NADA is the National Acupuncture Detoxification Association, a nonprofit group that promotes acupuncture as an adjunctive treatment for addiction and mental illness. NADA developed what is known as the Five Needle Protocol, abbreviated as 5NP: five needles placed in acupuncture points in the ear which alleviate the symptoms of drug and alcohol detoxification and which also reduce stress, anxiety, and depression. 5NP reduces cravings, improves sleep, diminishes drug dreams, increases energy, lowers blood pressure, and generally helps people in recovery stay centered.

The radical genius of NADA is how this treatment is provided: drug counselors, nurses, and other recovery professionals *who are not necessarily licensed acupuncturists* receive a 70 hour training to be certified as Acupuncture Detoxification Specialists, which means being able to put needles in people's ears. 5NP is an elegant, universally useful treatment which can be affordably provided to clients in recovery programs because the people who are offering the acupuncture already work in those programs, and they do not need to "become acupuncturists" before they can serve people with acupuncture.

The Chinese medical theory behind 5NP is readily accessible to laypersons within the 70 hour training; it is not cumbersome, and does not require a Chinese medical diagnostic process before it can be used. Virtually everyone can benefit from 5NP. Furthermore, NADA treatment is often delivered in silence -- no talking and no questions needed -- and almost always in a group setting, with patients sitting quietly in a circle for half an hour or so, receiving auricular acupuncture.

NADA's example shaped our understanding of how to set up our kitchen, in several important ways. First, there are some basic acupuncture protocols which are always beneficial to everyone, and that do not need to be modified to individuals. This means that a Chinese medical diagnosis is not always appropriate or useful -- which helped us fundamentally to separate acupuncture practice from acupuncture theory. Most people are suffering from qi not moving, and they need acupuncture, any acupuncture: that's the right "diagnosis". Second, treating multiple patients together in the same room is much more powerful than treating individuals in individual cubicles. There is a tangible calmness and peace that arises from patients sitting quietly getting acupuncture together, no matter who they are or what relationship they have to each other. If one of the definitions of qi is "atmosphere", there is a lot more qi moving when patients get acupuncture together than when they get it individually; it's not an easy concept to explain, but it's something that is easy to feel, when it's happening. Think "warm hum", multiplied and shared.

NADA's reach is often constrained by issues of funding. Many people who benefit from NADA style treatment are members of the underclass: not only suffering from addiction but chronically homeless or in prison. As a result, NADA programs generally depend on government support, grants or donations to provide acupuncture. These sources are unfortunately not always a stable foundation, since people suffering from addiction are rarely a high priority in terms of funding. For many clients who graduate from treatment, what happens is that, by means of hard internal work and enormous courage, they elevate themselves out of the underclass into the working class; instead of sleeping under bridges and getting high, they get a minimum-wage job and a cheap apartment and a new life in recovery. Sobriety is a hero's journey, but unfortunately, these heroes don't get acupuncture anymore; once they become working class, they generally no longer qualify for government funded treatment. Which means that just when they could use acupuncture more than ever -- when they are working at physically grueling jobs, making the transition out of the support and structure of a treatment program, trying to navigate a difficult life without turning to drugs -- they can't get any acupuncture, just because instead of having no money at all, they now have very little. These people represent the target patients for the community acupuncture business model.

Oh, If Only We Ruled the World: Acupuncture Education

Acupuncture students and prospective acupuncture students very often ask us for advice about education. And so as part of explaining how we set up our kitchen, we would like to describe how we wish that we had been trained to cook, and how we wish that we could train others to cook. Our Japanese acupuncture teacher, Yoshi Ikeda, liked to say that the practice of acupuncture requires you to develop your heart, your hands, and your head -- in that order of importance. He also liked to say that American acupuncture schools got it exactly backward, with students spending all their time in their heads.

If we were in charge of our future employees' acupuncture education, we would begin by asking them, before they cracked a book, to take the 70 hour NADA Acupuncture Detoxification Specialist training. Once they were qualified to use 5NP auricular acupuncture, we would see that they treated as many people as possible. Learning a simple protocol such as 5NP allows the student to focus on the heart skill of establishing rapport with patients and the hand skills of needling, without being distracted by a lot of head stuff.

Our next step would be to teach more needling skills. Doing ear acupuncture is significantly different than doing acupuncture in other places on the body, and acupuncture is a tactile, physical skill. It requires lots of practice, unencumbered by theory. In our kitchen, we use relatively fine needles (38 gauge Acuzone brand, mostly one inch), and some acupuncturists find that they take some getting used to.

Ah, but which points should these hypothetical students practice on? In most acupuncture schools, students spend their first year learning the locations of all 500 generally recognized points, even though they will never use most of them. We would prefer to have students immediately learn to needle just a few points, those that they would be most likely to use in the future.

If we were in charge of our future employees' acupuncture education, the next thing we would do would be to ask them to read one very short, lovely little book: Miriam Lee's <u>Insights of a Senior Acupuncturist</u>,[5] in which she describes how she dealt with the challenge of needing to treat as many as 17 patients an hour by creating a protocol of just five acupuncture points that could treat virtually everything. These would be the five points that we asked students to learn to needle first, since these are points which they can expect to use over and over, with great results, for decades. What is the reason for students to memorize 500 points, when only five could begin to teach them the very core of an effective practice? (And what are those five points? We're getting to that, we promise.)

A beginning cook should learn to scramble eggs before he tackles a soufflé. Similarly, there is very little practical value in having a beginning cook spend hours outside of a kitchen reading extensively about the intricacies of soufflés. A beginning acupuncturist should learn how to needle, memorize a few points, and practice the hell out of them before trying to learn any acupuncture theory. If you master some basic needling skills and you use fine needles, you are not going to hurt anyone with acupuncture. It's actually really difficult to hurt someone with acupuncture, and real injury generally requires misusing acupuncture points that we are not even going to discuss. If you choose to learn more acupuncture theory, it will be infinitely easier to do so within a context of practical experience.

At this point, if you are an interested patient or a new acupuncture student, we realize that it is possible that you are thinking, but *where, oh where* can I learn more about acupuncture theory?!? You may feel that you really just can't go any further into this discussion without some help in that regard. Okay. There are some books, obviously not including this one, that will be of assistance: <u>The Healing Power of Acupressure and Acupuncture</u> by Matthew Bauer is a good place for the layperson to begin to understand Chinese medical theory. <u>Who Can Ride the Dragon? An Exploration of the Cultural Roots of Traditional Chinese Medicine</u>, and <u>A Brief History of Qi</u>, by Zhang Yu Huan and Ken Rose, address acupuncture theory within the context of Chinese culture, religion and language. Finally, Richard Tan's <u>Acupuncture 1, 2, 3</u> summarizes the theoretical foundations of his very effective treatment methods. All of these books are concise and readable, even if you have little or no background in Chinese medicine.

For patients who just want a simple introduction to what we do, however, and for acupuncturists who are interested in the specifics of our clinical practice, however, here is a list of the acupuncture points that we use the most often, and a list of the recipes in which we use them.

Points/Ingredients

The most, well, comprehensive description of acupuncture points and their locations can be found in that weighty tome known as <u>Acupuncture: a Comprehensive Text</u>, from the Shanghai College of Traditional Medicine, edited by John O'Connor and Dan Bensky. A page-turner it is not, so for those of you who are just hoping to get a general overview, we are providing our own diagrams. If you are a patient, you should know that all of the points that we refer to have lovely, poetic Chinese names, but like most American acupuncturists, we don't refer to them by those names. Most points have a shorter designation consisting of the name of the meridian on which they are located, plus a number (for example, "Large Intestine 4"), and that is the designation that we use. We suggest that you think of this designation as the street address of the acupuncture point.

(What, you ask, is a meridian --also known as a channel? Alas, that is beyond the scope of this book. Meridians are very interesting and definitely worth learning about; the theory books we mentioned above can help you with that. For the purposes of our discussion, please think of the meridian as just the street where the acupuncture point lives. You will note that some of the points or point groups we list below simply have names, such as Yin Tang. Think of those like the addresses of rural country estates in English mystery novels, like "Hazelmoor", or "The Hollow" – you get the idea.)

In no particular order of importance, the main points that we use at Working Class Acupuncture, the ones we could get by with (and we think you could, too!) if every other acupuncture point somehow disappeared, are:

Large Intestine 4 and 11, Lung 7, Spleen 6, and Stomach 36 (these are Miriam Lee's five points that she describes in <u>Insights of a Senior Acupuncturist</u>).

Large Intestine 4 is such a geographically large point that it is really more of a zone than a point. We often describe it as LI 4, LI 4.5, and LI 3.5.

Similarly for Stomach 36. When we use this point, we often include multiple points between Stomach 36 and Stomach 39.

We'll discuss Intestine 4 and Stomach 36 more in "Needling in Clusters" below.

Liver 3 and 8
Gallbladder 40 and 34
Kidney 3 and 6
Bladder 60, 62, 64, and 65

Small Intestine 3, 3.5 (aka Shang Hou Xi), 4, and 6
Heart 3, 4, 5, 6, 7, and 8
Lung 5 and 10
Spleen 6, 8, and 9
Spleen 4 and Pericardium 6
Triple Warmer 5 and Gallbladder 41
Conception Vessel 6, 12, 17, and 22
Stomach 25, 40
Large Intestine 20
Bladder 7
Governing Vessel 20 and 24
Yin Tang
Si Shen Cong
Yao Tong
Luo Zhen
Ze Xia
NADA 5 Needle Protocol

That's it, that's the list.

Now we can practically hear the howls of outrage from certain acupuncturists and acupuncture students. **That's your list?** *Where are the back-shu points? How can you possibly do acupuncture without the back-shu points?* For those of you who don't know what all the ruckus is about, there are some very nice points on the back of the body known as back-shu points, which in our clinic we almost never use because almost all of our patients receive acupuncture sitting up in recliners rather than lying face down on a massage table. Some acupuncturists are very attached to the back-shu points, to the degree that they feel a treatment is not complete unless it includes points on the front and the back of the body. All we can say is that we like the back-shu points too, but we don't really miss them. We don't need them. We get good results without them, and we think you can too. There is no one right way to do acupuncture, remember?

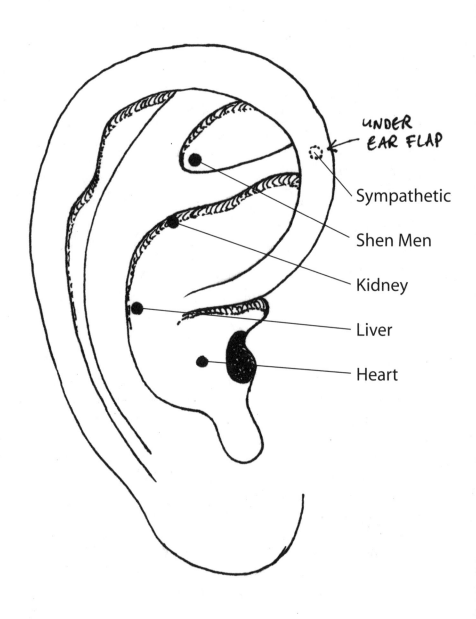

**The NADA 5NP
(5 Needle Protocol)**

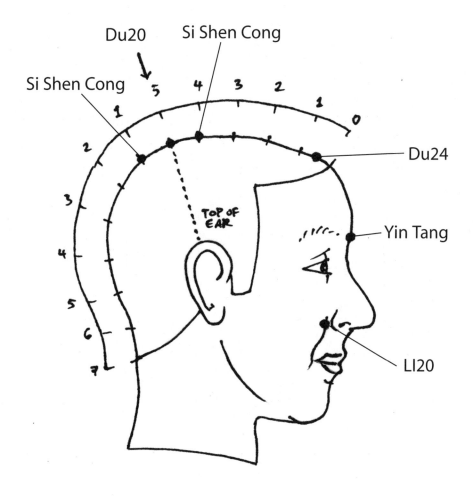

Major Acupuncture Points on the Head (Side View)

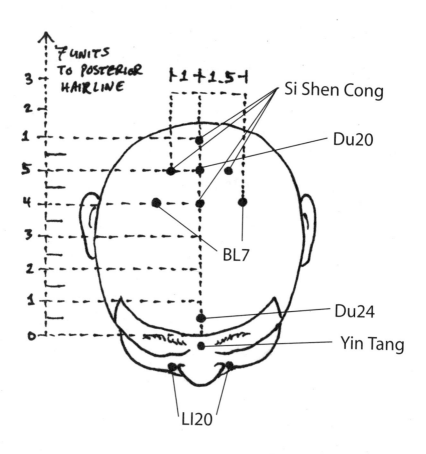

Major Acupuncture Points on the Head (Top View)

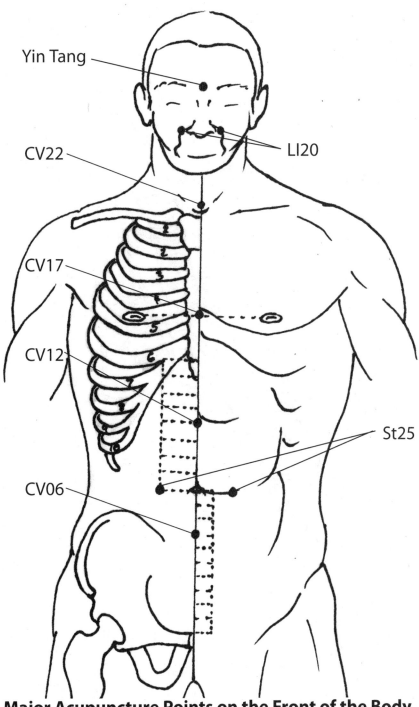

Major Acupuncture Points on the Front of the Body

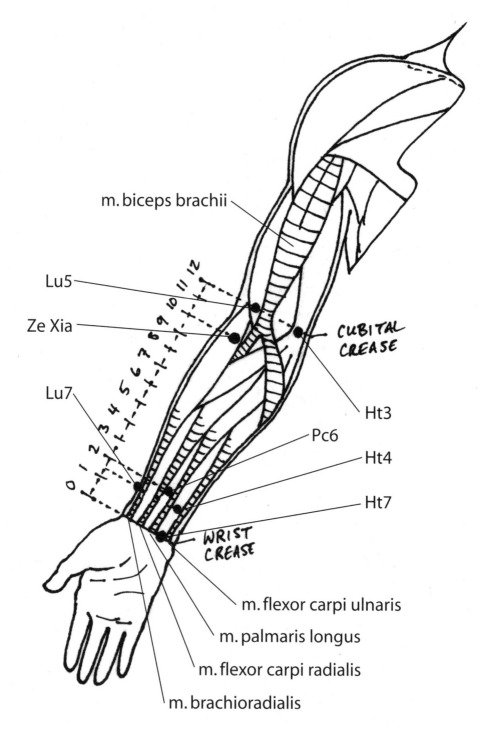

Major Acupuncture Points on the Arm

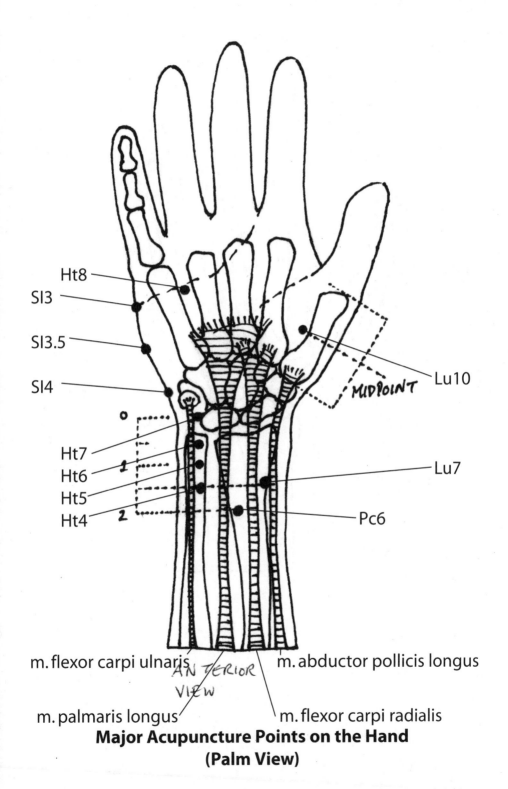

**Major Acupuncture Points on the Hand
(Palm View)**

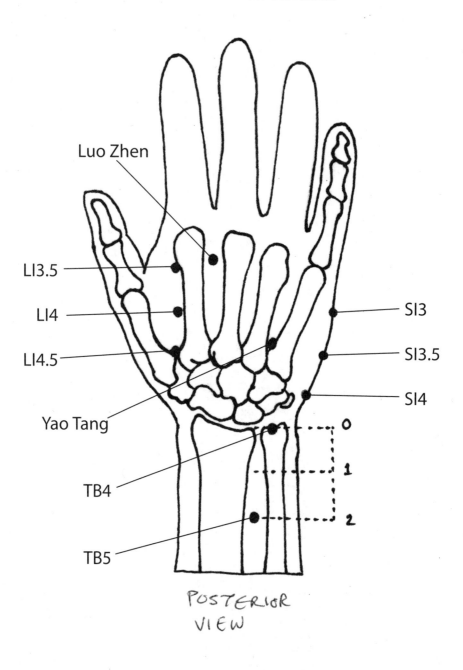

Major Acupuncture Points on the Hand (Back View)

Part Two: Welcome to Our Kitchen 45

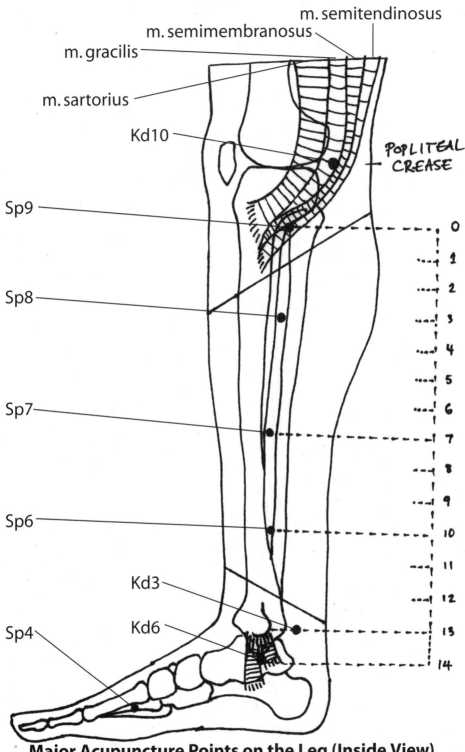

Major Acupuncture Points on the Leg (Inside View)

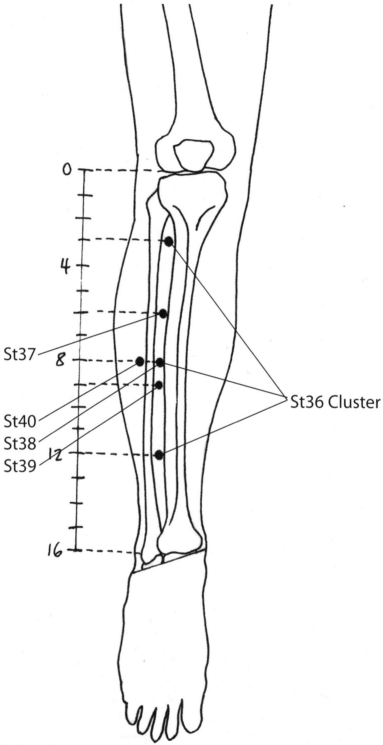

Major Acupuncture Points on the Leg (Front View)

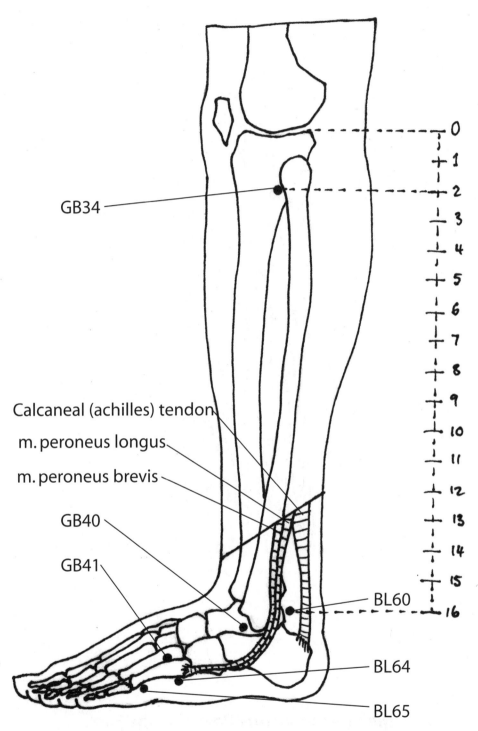

Major Acupuncture Points on the Leg (Side View)

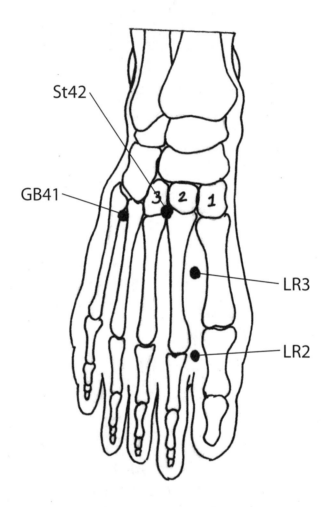

Major Acupuncture Points on the Foot

How We Treat Pain

For those people who are still howling – *but what about back pain? How can you possibly treat back pain without the back shu points?* We'll explain this in a minute, we promise. But we want to explain something else first, because our approach will make more sense that way. So hold off on the howling for a page or two, okay?

How We Treat Conditions Other Than Pain

Due to some acupuncture theory which we really like (yes, even we find acupuncture theory interesting) but really can't explain in this context, the points Liver 3 and Gallbladder 40 end up in 70% of the treatments we do. The best partial explanation we have, without quoting Chapter 9 of the Nei Jing Ling Shu, is that most Americans are really stressed out and specifically really need those points, because those points focus on the particular type of stress that most Americans have. What Liver 3 and Gallbladder 40 represent is very often that first domino that you need to knock over. You do not need to read Chapter 9 of the Nei Jing Ling Shu in order to verify the truth of this statement; just try adding those points to every treatment and see the results. As for the rest of the population, 20% of them will hugely benefit from the points Kidney 3 and Bladder 64, and about 10% need Spleen 3 and Stomach 42. But if you just needle Liver 3 and Gallbladder 40 on everyone, you'll help most people, and anyway, those are great points.[6]

As Miriam Lee explains so beautifully in her book, the points LI 4 and 11, Lu 7, Sp 6 and St 36 in combination are effective for virtually everything.[7] *If you want to make simple noodles for lots of people, approach the process of cooking by focusing on the* **commonalities** *rather than the* **differences** *between people.* Look for the points that help everybody with everything! We do this by having a "base" for many of our treatments, just as cooks make stock as a base for soups and sauces. Our soup stock is this combination of points:

Large Intestine 4 and 11, Lung 7, Spleen 6, Stomach 36, Gallbladder 40 and Liver 3, or (LI 4 & 11, Lu 7, Sp 6, St36, GB40, Liv 3)

and then we add more symptomatic points to that base. Like this:

Fatigue and/or "general maintenance": (LI 4 & 11, Lu 7, Sp 6, St36, GB40, Liv 3)

Strengthen immune system: (LI 4 & 11, Lu 7, Sp 6, St36, GB40, Liv 3)

Stress and/or anxiety: (LI 4 & 11, Lu 7, Sp 6, St36, GB40, Liv 3) plus 5NP, GV20 &24, Yin Tang

Stop Smoking: (LI 4 & 11, Lu 7, Sp 6, St36, GB40, Liv 3) plus 5 NP

Depression: (LI 4 & 11, Lu 7, Sp 6, St36, GB40, Liv 3) plus GB 34, St 40, Ht 7, Si Shen Cong

Digestive problems: (LI 4 & 11, Lu 7, Sp 6, St36, GB40, Liv 3) plus CV 12 & 6, St 25. Cluster needle St 36.

Sinusitis, allergies, and/or common cold: (LI 4 & 11, Lu 7, Sp 6, St36, GB40, Liv 3) plus LI 20, Bl7, Yin Tang

Flu: (LI 4 & 11, Lu 7, Sp 6, St36, GB40, Liv 3) plus TW 5 and GB 41

Sore throat: (LI 4 & 11, Lu 7, Sp 6, St36, GB40, Liv 3) plus CV 22, Lu 10

Cough: (LI 4 & 11, Lu 7, Sp 6, St36, GB40, Liv 3) plus CV 22, Lu 5, St 40

Diabetes: (LI 4 & 11, Lu 7, Sp 6, St36, GB40, Liv 3) plus Sp7, 8 and 9

Side effects of chemotherapy: (LI 4 & 11, Lu 7, Sp 6, St36, GB40, Liv 3) plus GV 20, Pc 6

Insomnia: (LI 4 & 11, Lu 7, Sp 6, St36, GB40, Liv 3) plus Ht 7, GV 20, 24, Yin Tang

Nightmares: (LI 4 & 11, Lu 7, Sp 6, St36, GB40, Liv 3) plus Ht 7, GV 20, 24, Yin Tang, Si Shen Cong

PMS: (LI 4 & 11, Lu 7, Sp 6, St36, GB40, Liv 3) plus SP4, Pc 6/ or TW 5, GB41

Infertility: (LI 4 & 11, Lu 7, Sp 6, St36, GB40, Liv 3) plus Kid 6 and SP4, Pc 6/ or TW 5, GB41

Anything so complicated that you think you don't even know where to start: (LI 4 & 11, Lu 7, Sp 6, St36, GB40, Liv 3)

Are you getting the idea here? See how simple this can be? If you're still not convinced, go read Miriam Lee's book and then come back.

Unilateral/Bilateral

We have found that we get good results doing either unilateral or bilateral treatments. The things we like about unilateral treatments are that they save needles. Certain sensitive patients particularly appreciate their acupuncturist saving needles. What this means in plain English is: you don't have to use all of the points in a recipe on both sides of the body, and there are no absolute rules about how to choose which points go where. Here are some examples.

You can use our "soup stock" recipe like this, alternating yin and yang points:

Left arm: LI 4, LI 11
Right arm: Lu 7
Left leg: Liv 3, Sp 6
Right leg: St 36, GB 40

Or like this, not alternating yin and yang points but still saving needles:

Left arm: LI 4, Lu 7
Right arm: LI 4, LI 11
Left leg: Liv 3, Sp 6, GB 40
Right leg: St 36, Liv 3, GB 40

In our experience, it works just as well either way. We typically try to make the unilateral treatments look roughly symmetrical (two points on each arm, three points on each leg, etc.), because we like symmetry. We have never tried doing a wildly asymmetrical treatment, such as doing all of the points on only one side of the body, so we can't recommend that; we don't like how it looks and we don't know if it would work. But, acupuncture being what it is, it very well might work just as well as anything else.

Okay, Now We Will Explain How We Treat Pain

Pain is what most acupuncture clinics treat most often, and our clinic is no exception. What non-acupuncturists need to know before reading this section is that acupuncturists tend to rely on two basic strategies for treating pain: local treatment and distal treatment. Local treatment means that you put needles where the pain is; treating back pain requires that you needle the back. (That's what prompted all that howling a few pages ago.) Distal treatment means that you put needles somewhere other than where the pain is; for example, a distal treatment for back pain might rely primarily on needles in the hand. Distal treatment for pain has gotten a huge boost in the acupuncture world in the last decade or so thanks to the work of Dr. Richard Tan, who created what he calls "the Balance Method". Acupuncturists who rely on distal treatments for pain sometimes quarrel with acupuncturists who rely on local treatments for pain about which is most effective, and the underlying theories. However, our description of how we treat pain in our clinic is probably going to mortally offend both acupuncturists who rely on local treatment AND acupuncturists who rely on distal treatment.[8]

Why is that? Because how we treat pain has nothing to do with acupuncture theory.

As we mentioned before, even we like acupuncture theory. The acupuncture theory we like most is known as Jingei Pulse Diagnosis, an obscure method of pulse diagnosis based on an ancient Chinese medical classic known as the Nei Jing Ling Shu. We learned Jingei from Yoshi Ikeda, the talented Japanese acupuncturist who told us to develop our hearts, hands, and heads, in that order. Some aspects of how we treat pain have to do with the theories behind Jingei Pulse Diagnosis, but – here's the kicker – you don't need to understand anything about Jingei Pulse Diagnosis to use our methods. You just need to follow our recipes. They will work just fine.[9]

Similarly, we like Richard Tan's Balance Method. We think it's neat; we have experimented with some of his points and point combinations, and they work. We like his books, especially Twelve and Twelve in Acupuncture and Twenty–Four More.[10] We regularly encourage acupuncturists, especially those who lack clinical confidence, to buy his books and attend his seminars. However, the Balance Method is a set of theories, and it has rules. We have noticed lots of acupuncturists becoming preoccupied with how to follow the orthodoxies of the Balance Method, but we are not convinced that orthodox Balance Method acupuncturists get any better results clinically than heretical pragmatists like us. We do not believe that following theoretical rules is ever the point of practicing acupuncture. Furthermore, some acupuncturists believe that the only effective way to treat pain with distal points is the Balance Method, and this simply isn't true. You can treat many common types of pain perfectly well simply by using the points on the list we gave you above. All of those are points and indications found in Acupuncture: a Comprehensive Text, which is a basic TCM (Traditional Chinese Medicine, aka Acupuncture Organized by Communist Bureaucrats) reference book. You don't need theories to treat pain, either; you can just follow recipes.

All you acupuncturists can resume the outraged howling any time now – don't feel you have to wait until we list the recipes.

Needling In Clusters

One of the odd things we do in our clinic, besides treating people in a common space and ignoring acupuncture theory of all varieties, is that we often needle acupuncture points in little clusters: meaning, instead of putting one needle in a point, we will put three or four needles together in a little group. We don't know why we do this; we started doing it many years ago, and it just looked right, so we kept doing it. Practicing acupuncture is sometimes kind of like arranging flowers. We learned much later about another famous acupuncturist, the great Master Tung, who also puts needles in groups of three. Master Tung has his own unique set of acupuncture points and his own acupuncture theories, which – can you guess? We also like, and we know they work, but no, we are not followers of Master Tung and we don't really care about his theories, either. We thought it was really nifty when we found out that Master Tung needled in groups of three, but if Master Tung were alive to see how we've been doing it, he would probably be horrified at the haphazardness of it all.[11]

We use a lot of "cluster needles" when we treat pain, so we wanted to explain this first. We have no real method about how we decide how to space the needles in a cluster; it just has to look right and feel right to us.

A Few Pain Recipes, with Explanations

Low back pain, also known as the number one reason to see an acupuncturist.

Bilateral: Yao Tong, LI 4 (cluster points), SI 6, 4, 3.5, and 3 (which is also basically a cluster, although SI 3.5 happens to have its own name, Shanghouxi); GB 40, 34; Bl 60, 62, 64, 65; Kid 3, Liv 3, GV 20

Unilateral, left sided low back pain: GV 20
Left arm: Ze Xia, Lu 10 (cluster)
Right arm: LI 4(cluster) SI 4, 3.5, and 3, Yao Tong, TW 5
Right leg: Liv 3, Kid 3
Left leg: GB 40, 34; Bl 60, 62, 64, 65
Unilateral, right sided low back pain: reverse above
Explanation: Lu 10, LI 4, SI 6, 4, 3.5, and 3, and Yao Tong all have traditional (TCM) indications either for back pain specifically or for all pain in general (LI 4). Ze Xia is a point that we have found very useful for back

pain. The use of paired source points (Liv 3 and GB 40, Kid 3 and Bl 64) comes from Jingei Pulse Diagnosis. GB 34 and the other Bladder points have traditional indications for back pain (as does Kid 3). We would use Bl 40, behind the knee, as well, but it's sometimes hard to reach in a recliner. With a little practice you can feel the point with one hand while the other slides the needle and guide tube under the knee, then insert the needle so that it is parallel to the cushion of the chair. (Don't worry, the angle is very oblique, but you will still be stimulating the point.) We think GV 20 is a good point for anything having to do with the spine.

Upper back pain

Bilateral: Lu 10 (cluster,) Yao Tong, TW 5; GB 40, 34; Bl 60, 62, 64, 65; Kid 3, Liv 3, GV 20
    Unilateral, left sided upper back pain: GV 20
    Right arm: Ze Xia, Lu 10 (cluster)
    Left arm: LI 4(cluster) SI 6, 4, 3.5, and 3, Yao Tong, TW 5
    Left leg: Liv 3, Kid 3
    Right leg: GB 40, 34; Bl 60, 62, 64, 65
    Unilateral, right sided upper back pain: reverse above
    Explanation: see explanation for low back pain, above. We tend to think of the Lu 10 cluster as more specifically useful for upper back pain (because that's where the lungs are?), although it is traditionally indicated for all back pain, and so we emphasize it over the LI 4 cluster in this recipe. TW 5 is traditionally indicated for stiff necks, but we think it works for all back pain, especially upper back pain.

Neck pain

Also including the area of the trapezius (some patients will refer to this as "shoulder pain", so you have to ask them where it hurts):
Unilateral OR Bilateral: GV 20
    Left arm: Heart 4, 5, 6, 7 (cluster)
    Right arm: SI 6, 4, 3.5, and 3, Luo Zhen, TW 5
    Right leg: Liv 3, Kid 3
    Left leg: GB 40, 34; Bl 60, 62, 64, 65
Explanation: Pairing the source points of Ht 7 and SI 4 comes from Jingei Pulse Diagnosis. Since we cluster needles around SI 4, however, we do the same with Ht 7 (those points are very close together anyway). Luo Zhen and TW 5 are traditionally indicated for stiff necks. The explanation for the leg points are the same as above, for back pain; it's a combination of Jingei Pulse Diagnosis

and our belief that all of those lower Bladder points work on the spine. And as for why we have the same recipe for unilateral or bilateral neck pain? If you look at the locations for the clusters of needles around SI4 and Ht 7, you can see that it would be pretty hard to needle both of those clusters on the same hand. So even if the pain is bilateral, the needles are unilateral – it works just as well.

Knee pain

(LI 4 & 11, Lu 7, Sp 6, St36, GB40, Liv 3) plus Kid 10, Sp 9, Liv 8, and GB 34. We suggest doing cluster needles on LI 4 and on LI 11. The treatment looks better that way. (But we do not encourage anyone to cluster needle anywhere around Lu 7, ever, because there isn't enough flesh on most people there and it will just hurt.) It doesn't matter if the pain is unilateral or bilateral.

Shoulder pain

It's very important to find out what people mean when they say "shoulder pain", as they may mean trapezius, upper back, or arm pain. In this treatment we are referring to pain mostly in the shoulder joint, but we include points that will help with the upper back as well.
Bilateral: SI 6 and 4, TW 5, GB 34, 40, 41, ST 38 (cluster), Sp 8 and 9 (cluster), Liv 3

>Unilateral, left sided shoulder pain:
>Left arm: Lu 10 (cluster)
>Right arm: SI 6 and 4, TW 5
>Right leg: SP 8 and 9 cluster, Liv 3
>Left leg: GB 34, 40, 41, St 38 cluster
>Unilateral, right sided shoulder pain: reverse above

SI 6 and TW 5 are traditionally indicated for shoulder pain. TW 5 together with GB 41 treats joint pain in general. Liv 3, GB 40 and GB 34 originate with Jingei Pulse Diagnosis, and address the tendons. St 38 is traditionally indicated for shoulder inflammation, but we have found through trial and error that cluster needling around Sp 8 and Sp 9 works in a very similar way.

Headache: Frontal

(LI 4 & 11, Lu 7, Sp 6, St36, GB40, Liv 3) plus Sp 9, Lu 10, and Ht 3. If the headache is intense, try cluster needling Sp 9 and St 36. This works especially well for sinus headaches.

Headache: Vertex

(LI 4 & 11, Lu 7, Sp 6, St36, GB40, Liv 3) plus Ht 3, Lu 10, and GB 34.

Headache: Occiput

See: "Neck Pain"; add Ht 3 to the other Heart points.

Headache: Left Temporal

>Left arm: LI 4, TW 5
>Right arm: Ht 8, Ht 3
>Right leg: GB 34, 40, 41, Bl 64
>Left leg: Liv 3, Liv 8, Sp 4

Headache: Right Temporal

Reverse above.
Explanation: Ht 3 is traditionally indicated for headaches. We have found that Lu 10 and Ht 8 work well also, though Lu 10 works better for frontal headaches, and Ht 8 works better for temporal headaches.

Cooking: Get the Needles in the Patients with a Minimum of Fuss and Then Leave Them In as Long as They Want. And Repeat.

Noodles are made out of flour; acupuncture treatments are made out of concentrated stillness.

Unfortunately, many conventional acupuncturists are not primarily practicing acupuncture. They are prescribing herbs, or doing lifestyle counseling, or lecturing their patients about nutrition, with a little acupuncture on the side. Often this is because they don't really believe that acupuncture, all by itself, really works. And often this is because they have never used acupuncture the way it was meant to be used, with patients receiving it frequently and regularly; they have never gotten satisfactory clinical results, so they don't think satisfactory clinical results are even possible with acupuncture alone. As a result, instead of doing acupuncture, what they are really doing is a whole lot of talking.

As unkind as this is, the easiest way to understand many of our clinic's kitchen procedures is to look at how acupuncture schools teach students how to do acupuncture -- and then do the exact opposite. For instance, an acupuncture treatment at most acupuncture school clinics consists of at least half an hour of talking to the patient, between asking questions and giving (usually unsolicited) lifestyle advice, and then only ten to twenty minutes of the patient resting in silence with the needles. Michael Smith, the founder of NADA, describes this as "front-loading" a treatment, and just thinking about it makes us unhappy. Patients who have experienced this kind of acupuncture sometimes describe it like this: "they asked me all of these really weird questions before they treated me, and then just when I was starting to relax into it and feel really good, they took out the needles and made me get up and leave."

Our perspective is that the most important part of any acupuncture treatment happens after the acupuncturist puts in the last needle and walks away. What happens inside the patient, while he or she is sitting in silence with the needles, is what does the real work. Everything else, including everything the acupuncturist does and says, should be an unobtrusive support to that central silence.

Let's consider first the issue of the "patient intake". Conventional acupuncturists believe that they need to ask lots of questions before they can start putting the needles in. This would make sense if designing an acupuncture treatment were like prescribing a drug; obviously there's a big difference between an antipsychotic and an antibiotic, and you'd better not confuse them. But when you look at how acupuncture really works, in the clinic, with real people, there is not necessarily a lot of difference between a treatment for mental illness and a treatment for physical illness. Remember that continuum of a human being? All of the points have so many different functions, there is in fact no way to even know what each point might be doing for a given patient in a particular treatment. In our experience, some acupuncture points are certainly more effective than others for certain problems (that's why we gave you a list), but any point is most likely going to do something useful.

This gets back to the issue of acupuncture being like noodles. If someone came to you and said he was hungry, and you happened to have a bowl of noodles readily available, we hope that what you would do is smile at the person and give him the noodles. It would be very odd if you insisted on spending half an hour interrogating the person before you fed him. "Oh, so how long have you felt hungry? Have you ever been hungry before? On a scale of one to ten, how hungry are you? Does your hunger feel sharp or dull? Do you feel the hunger deep in the pit of your stomach, or are you just a little peckish? Is anyone else in your family hungry? Were you breast fed as a baby? Did your family ever have fights at the dinner table? Do you think you might have some unresolved emotional issues about food?" Etc, etc, etc.

This kind of interrogation makes no sense if you are serving food rather than prescribing pharmaceuticals. No matter what your patient says, at the end of it all you will just be giving him acupuncture. You may change the flavor of the acupuncture you are giving him by selecting slightly different points, but all you can do is change the flavor, you can't make what you have to offer into something more complex than a bowl of noodles. Furthermore, you cannot control your patient's process of digestion; we have observed many times that the exact same set of points will have a different result in different patients, or different results in the same patient on different days. Acupuncture is initiating processes inside the body that no acupuncturist can fully comprehend -- so we strongly encourage you to just shut up already and get the needles in the patient, and have faith that something good will happen if you do.

In our previous lives before we discovered the community acupuncture model, we used to spend a long time asking patients questions because we, too, had been convinced that this somehow made us "responsible". After a few years of this, it began to dawn on us that no matter what the patient said, it had little or no impact on which acupuncture points we chose. One of the only really meaningful questions for an acupuncturist, in terms of point selection, is "where does it hurt?" The answer to that question can make a difference in whether or not a treatment is effective; answers to virtually every other possible question, however, don't.

Similarly, one of the lessons we learned from watching how effective the simple NADA auricular protocol can be, is that the process many acupuncturists use of carefully manipulating the needles in order to "tonify" or "disperse" the acupuncture points is largely overrated. We have found that just putting the needles in works wonders -- provided that you leave them in long enough. We do try to "get qi", meaning that we want the patient to feel that something is happening. And then we get out of the way, literally and figuratively.

One of the most distinctive elements to our kitchen, or our clinical operations, is that we believe that patients should keep the needles in until they feel that they are "cooked", and that they should tell the acupuncturist when they are done rather than the acupuncturist telling them. Virtually every patient, with a little bit of practice, can learn to feel when the process of an acupuncture treatment is complete, when everything that is going to happened has already happened, and it's time to take the needles out. This time period varies enormously from person to person, but in general is much, much longer than most conventional acupuncturists believe.

Many acupuncturists think that leaving the needles in more than ten to twenty minutes can "drain" a person, leaving them tired and feeling worse than before. Our observations suggest the contrary: the vast majority of patients get infinitely better clinical results when they are allowed to stay as long as they want, which can include falling into a deep, restful sleep and then waking up naturally. Some patients stay for hours and wake feeling happy and refreshed. The average "cooking time" for most people tends to be around an hour.

We also recommend that patients get acupuncture much more frequently and regularly than most conventional acupuncturists. Figuring out how often a patient should come is the one place that we use pain scales. If a condition is acute (such as a recently sprained ankle) or the pain is intense (above an 8 on a scale of 1 to 10), we recommend that the patient get acupuncture every day for at least five days. If a patient says her pain is 10 on a scale of 10, we recommend she get acupuncture every day until the pain decreases significantly. For problems that are less intense but still troublesome, we recommend that patients get acupuncture two to three times a week. To maintain a person who has gotten better but is not yet out of the woods -- say, a barista with wrist problems who has to keep making coffee for a living -- we recommend weekly treatments. In general, when we set up a treatment plan with a patient, we recommend six to ten treatments in a row at suitable intervals. For chronic, severe problems, we tell patients that they will probably need regular treatment for months. And of course, many patients get acupuncture on a regular or semi-regular basis just because they enjoy it so much.

How Our Treatment Room Looks and Why

The most visibly unusual aspect of our kitchen is our treatment space itself. Most acupuncture treatment settings (apart from NADA programs) are structured around a basic unit: one cubicle, one massage table, one patient, one hour. These units may be multiplied (several cubicles, several patients) but the basic structure remains the same. The basic unit of the community acupuncture model is: one large room, multiple recliners, four to six patients an hour per acupuncturist, and many concurrent naps.

We treat patients in community. That's why we call it community acupuncture. We're not going to go in to how it evolved,[12] except to thank NADA once again for the inspiration; we're just going to discuss how it works.

It comes as a big surprise to many acupuncturists that lots of patients actively prefer receiving acupuncture in recliners with other people around to receiving acupuncture alone in a little cubicle. Snoring does occasionally become an issue, but the simple solution is to ask people to bring earplugs. Otherwise, the benefits are numerous.

First, there is the "safety in numbers" benefit. Many patients who are nervous about acupuncture come in for the first time in the company of a friend or relative who is already a patient. They can sit next to each other, and the new patient can watch the returning patient getting acupuncture, so that it isn't so scary when it's their turn. On the same note, simply walking into a room full of deeply relaxed people makes new patients feel safer; they can look around and see that there is nothing to fear.

Second, the group setting makes it possible for patients to feel in control of their experience. Since an acupuncturist is always either treating someone or just walking through the room keeping an eye on everyone, it is easy for patients to signal that they are ready to get up because they feel "cooked". If we were to try to let patients time their own treatments in individual cubicles, we would have to be constantly opening and shutting the doors to check on them, and disturbing them in the process.

Third, the group setting keeps the focus on the acupuncture and off the talking. Many acupuncturists immediately panic about confidentiality issues in a group setting. However, confidentiality is much less of an issue if you are not asking people a series of intrusive questions. Most of what people suffer from does not require either analysis or discussion, and remember, you need very little information in order to choose acupuncture points that will work. Patient interviews in the community setting generally sound like this:

Acupuncturist (whispering): So? How's your back this week?
Patient (also whispering): I think it's better. I'm sleeping through the night.
Acupuncturist (whispering): Great! Is the pain still in the same place?
Patient (whispering): Yes.
Acupuncturist (whispering): OK. (Reaches for needles as a sign the conversation is complete).
Patient settles back and closes eyes. Acupuncturist gets to work.

And that's all, folks.
Even in the case of a mental/emotional issue, the conversation can sound like this:

Acupuncturist (whispering, having read patient's chart and knowing the chief complaint is depression): So how are you doing this week?
Patient (whispering): I felt really good after the last treatment for like, a whole day. And I think I might have a little more motivation.
Acupuncturist (whispering): And how's your sleep?
Patient (whispering): Not much change there.
Acupuncturist (whispering): OK. (Reaches for needles as a sign the conversation is complete).
Patient settles back and closes eyes. Acupuncturist gets to work.

Other patients in the room are probably asleep anyway; if they are not, and somehow overhear this conversation despite the white noise machines and the background music, they have not learned any private, compromising health information. A visiting acupuncturist once asked one of our long-term patients how he would feel about running into someone he knew at the clinic while he was getting acupuncture, and if that would make him uncomfortable. The patient looked at the acupuncturist in disbelief. "I'm coming in to get *acupuncture*. It's not like I'm walking in to a *crack house* or something." Patients don't feel pressured to say or do anything that would make them uncomfortable, so there is no problem with having other people around.

Fourth, the group setting makes it possible to keep interactions between patients and acupuncturists brief and efficient, which also helps patients to focus on themselves rather than on the acupuncturist. Many acupuncturists worry about patients going on and on about their problems and causing the acupuncturist to fall behind in the schedule. In reality, this doesn't happen, because patients are naturally considerate; they look around and see that other people are waiting to be treated, and so they get to the point. (Also, it's hard to go on and on about your problems in a whisper.) The presence of other patients who are focused inwardly helps new patients do the same. The group setting encourages patients to take responsibility for themselves, and so it has an empowering effect.

Fifth, "community qi" feels wonderful. It really does. Many patients say that just sitting down in a chair in this big, hushed room full of people getting acupuncture makes them feel better before they even get acupuncture themselves. "I like just hearing other people breathing," one of our patients said. It's similar to what happens when people do yoga together or meditate together or pray together; the collective stillness is palpable. "This is the most peaceful place in Portland," another patient said. (Which is saying a lot, we think, because Portland has some really nice public parks.) Most people who get acupuncture in community settings feel that the effect of the treatments is enhanced by having other people getting treated at the same time; they get better clinical results. They also feel that they are part of something larger than themselves, which even apart from the acupuncture, is soothing and uplifting. Although patients come in and get treated ten minutes apart, they will often synchronize their naps, so that sometimes everybody wakes up at once. A really strong napper can often pull a whole group of people down with him. When that happens, once they all wake up together, they tend to smile sleepily at each other as if they are all thinking, What happened there?

Community qi happened. Noodles taste better when you eat them with other people than when you eat them alone.

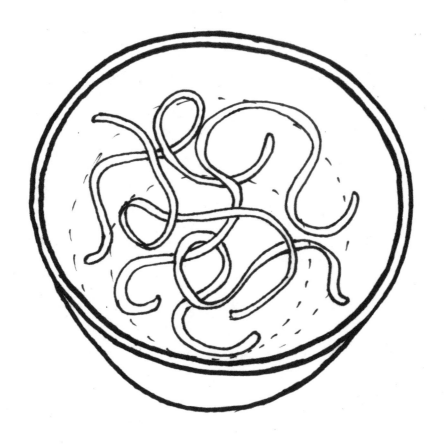

Part Three: Welcome to Our Dining Room (and Our Systems)

There is not a lot of point in being a talented chef if there is no one to eat the noodles you have so lovingly created. Many acupuncturists like to have endless debates about what style of acupuncture works best -- Traditional Chinese Medicine, Five Element, Toyohari, etc. -- but the reality is that NONE of those styles work at ALL unless the patient receives them in sufficient quantity. No treatment strategy works in reality if the patient doesn't stick with the treatment plan. At the moment, there are an awful lot of beautifully decorated acupuncture clinics with highly trained acupuncturists in America -- all sitting around anxiously staring at the phone, because there are no patients coming in. Who cares about what they know how to do, if they're not able to do it, because they have no one to do it with?

We do not believe that you can separate the efficacy of treatment from the cost of treatment. It doesn't matter what the academic arguments are for this style of acupuncture or that style of acupuncture; if you can't get the needles in the patient because the patient can't afford it, *then acupuncture doesn't work*. Everything about how we have set up our dining room is based on two complementary sets of concerns: the practical considerations of how to make the clinic finances support the clinic mission, and the larger desire for our business to reflect working class/lower middle class values like: *family connections, frugality, hard work, stability, simplicity, ease, interdependence, creativity, resourcefulness, personal relationships, directness, and loyalty*. The essence of the community acupuncture business model is that it is low-cost, high-volume, self-sustaining, and community based.

Low-cost, high volume means, first, that each acupuncture treatment costs between $15 and $35, and each patient decides what to pay on that scale each time he or she gets a treatment. The clinic needs to treat a lot of patients to sustain itself. However, low-cost, high-volume also means not just a high volume of individual patients, but a high volume of acupuncture treatments per patient, which in turn is made possible because of the low cost of each treatment. Acupuncture works best in quantity: either a lot of treatments, spaced very close together, over a short period of time for an acute condition, or a lot of treatments, spaced regularly apart, over a long period of time for a chronic condition.

We have had patients show up at our clinic who tell us that they love acupuncture, but because of the cost in conventional settings, they have been getting a treatment once every six weeks. (Like clockwork!) Those patients also tell us that, while they love the relaxation of the treatment while they're having it, the results don't last long. In other words, many conventional acupuncturists are operating a high-cost, very low-volume practice, which ends up with patients describing acupuncture like this: "well, it feels nice, but it sure costs a lot, and I guess it doesn't really do much". This is not the kind of reputation acupuncture needs, and it probably goes a long way towards explaining why so many acupuncture practices fail. On the other hand, the consequences of using a low-cost, high volume model for acupuncture are, first, excellent clinical results, because patients can afford to get enough acupuncture to make a difference; and, second, patients referring their family members and friends in large numbers. The community acupuncture business model, used correctly, creates a kind of endlessly renewing cycle of frequent, regular treatments; great results; and a high volume of patients, which each part of the cycle reinforcing the others.

What do we mean when we say that the community acupuncture business model is self-sustaining and community based? We mean that we depend on, and fully trust, this endlessly renewing cycle of inexpensive treatments, great results, and lots of patients. We do not seek any other means of support for the clinic. This means that we do not bill insurance, nor do we have any relationship with an insurance company. It also means that we do not seek other sources of funding, such as grants. And we do not charge some patients market rates for conventional acupuncture with the idea that those patients will somehow fund low cost treatments for everybody else. Our clinic has only one source of support, and that is our community of patients, all of whom are on an equal footing.

Portland, Oregon, where we live, is blessed with a large number of pho restaurants. Pho is Vietnamese noodle soup: rice noodles in an aromatic broth, garnished (or not) with meat, accompanied by a plate of fresh bean sprouts, basil, and chilies. You can get a huge bowl for about six dollars. You can find pho at a few high-end restaurants -- of course you can, it's delicious -- but most pho is served in very unpretentious settings that are notable for their basic decor and their ability to seat large family groups (think strip malls, fake plants, big round tables and plastic spoons). The basic menu never changes. A good pho restaurant is always full at all hours with all kinds of people: construction workers, executives on their lunch break, Vietnamese families with lots of little kids, all of them eating the same noodle soup. We want our dining room, the business of providing acupuncture, to feel like and function like a good pho restaurant: reliable, uncomplicated, social and nourishing.

A low-cost, high-volume practice requires not only a lot of patients, but also a lot of systems, to sustain itself. An acupuncturist who is seeing only a handful of patients, spending a great deal of time with each one, and charging each patient a lot of money, might be able to get by without systems; he or she could do something different with every patient, every time, and compensate for chaos with lots of individual attention. Our clinic, on the other hand, has six full time acupuncturists, each seeing around 70 patients each week. Like a busy restaurant, we can't tolerate inconsistency or chaos. We have had to develop an entire set of systems to make our clinic possible, and in the process we have become more and more enamored with our systems. The better they work, the more we love them, and the more we love them, the better they work. Systems are what our dining room is all about, because they are the foundation of our relationships with our community.

Our Basic Systems

This is what happens when a patient -- let's call her Maria -- comes to our clinic for acupuncture:

Maria walks in the door and is greeted by one of our receptionists. Maria hands the receptionist a $20 bill. "Would you like change?" the receptionist asks her. "No? Thank you very much. When would you like to come again?" Maria looks at her calendar, says, "how about the usual?" and the receptionist schedules another appointment for her at the same time next week. "OK, thank you! You can go ahead back!"

Maria walks back into the treatment area, stopping to thoughtfully switch off her cell phone. She finds her favorite recliner, sits down, and takes off her shoes and socks. She rolls her jeans up to just below her knees and pulls her sleeves up to her elbows. She finds the lever on the recliner under the fleece blanket that covers it, raises the lever and pushes back until she is in the position she likes, about half-way reclined. She closes her eyes and listens to the ambient music in the background.

After a few minutes, her acupuncturist pulls up one of the clinic's rolling stools next to Maria and sits down. "Hey, Maria", he says quietly. "What can I do for you today?"

"Oh, the usual -- my sinuses are really bothering me this week. Must be all the pollen. Otherwise I'm doing pretty good, my neck has been so much better since you treated me for it last time."

"Great," says her acupuncturist. He begins putting in needles. "Do you feel the sinus pressure just in your nose, or up in your forehead too?"

"Here," Maria says, "and here", pressing with her fingers on the spots that hurt. The acupuncturist puts more needles in.

"OK, are you comfortable? Do you need a blanket?" he asks when he's done.

"I'd love a blanket. Thank you very much." And Maria drifts off into a nap while her acupuncturist moves on to his next patient, who is just now sitting down across from Maria.

What makes our clinic successful is that this basic interaction is repeated some 450 times a week. These are the systems that make it possible:

1. The sliding scale, aka "community fee structure"

Maria is a grocery checker at Safeway. She gets acupuncture every week throughout the spring and fall to keep her seasonal sinusitis under control. She chooses to pay $20 per treatment, which she is able to commit to because she only needs to come once a week for three months at a time.

All of the patients at our clinic are offered the same sliding scale. We encourage them to pay what they feel comfortable with in order to fulfill the treatment plan that their acupuncturist suggests. Some patients pay the same fee every time; many pay more when they are able to. Some patients adjust their payment based on how often they are coming in; they often pay less at the beginning of treatment when they are coming in two or three times a week, and then pay more when they need less frequent treatments.

Many acupuncturists only think of a sliding scale fee structure in the context of charity clinics, where patients need to present income verification to qualify for reduced rates. This is not what we do. Our sliding scale is a form of customer service, and an acknowledgement of two basic realities: first, everybody needs acupuncture, but people's financial circumstances vary widely; and second, acupuncture only works if you get enough of it, and people will need varying amounts of it according to the nature and the severity of their problems. Our sliding scale is an effort to provide good customer service. We would never dream of requesting income verification -- otherwise known as "humiliating the patients by making them prove that they are poor enough to deserve our saintly generosity". That income verification is bad (very, very bad) customer service should be obvious to everyone.

New patients are sometimes taken aback by the idea that they get to choose how much they pay, but they generally adapt to the idea quickly once they understand the way that acupuncture works. Since the amount and frequency of treatment they need will vary, the amount of what they pay can vary too.

2. Reception, aka "the separation of money and treatment"

Many acupuncturists, because they do not see enough patients, never develop a system for taking money and scheduling. This quickly becomes an obstacle to having a high-volume practice, not least because having the same person giving the treatment and collecting the money gives rise to awkwardness. We separate the issues of money and treatment by hiring very competent receptionists, most of them retired women with stellar people skills.

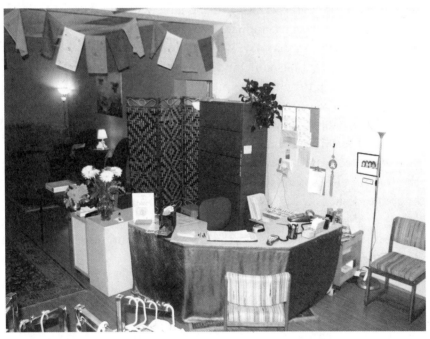

Working Class Acupuncture Reception Area

Our very first receptionist, Ilse Petesz, came up with the brilliant idea of teaching patients not only to pay for their treatment first, but also to schedule their next treatment before getting acupuncture. She observed that patients became so relaxed after getting acupuncture that they often drifted out the door in a blissful haze, forgetting to pay and unable to focus enough to schedule another treatment. Getting the business out of the way first is preferable for a variety of reasons; it's better for the clinic's cash flow, it reinforces the idea in everyone's minds that acupuncture is a process rather than a one-time occurrence, and it encourages the patients to let go of everything once they are settled in the treatment room -- once they leave the receptionist, there is nothing more that they will be needing their left brains for. Finally, it is a system, and so it takes away any awkwardness associated with money and payment by creating a consistent, impersonal process.

Another low cost system to separate money and treatment, also devised by a brilliant WCA employee, Lupine Hudson, is a system we call "the Invisible Receptionist". Lupine came up with the Invisible Receptionist to help other community acupuncture clinics that are not yet large enough to employ a human being to take care of reception.

The Invisible Receptionist works like this: when patients enter the clinic waiting room, they find a table where they can take care of their own payment, scheduling, and receipts. On the table will be a box with envelopes in it, the clinic schedule, a receipt pad, and a secure payment box. Each patient who has an appointment that day will find an open envelope in the envelope box marked with their first name and last initial. They put their payment in the envelope and drop the envelope into the secure payment box. If they forgot their checkbook or want to pay for a missed visit, they can put a note to that effect into the envelope. They schedule their next appointment by putting their first name and last initial into the schedule at their chosen time. They fill out their own receipts if they need them. Most acupuncturists have found that the Invisible Receptionist, while definitely not the same as having a real person at the desk, is a big improvement over trying to handle money and scheduling themselves at the same time that they are providing acupuncture. Some acupuncturists have adapted the Invisible Receptionist system to work with online scheduling.

3. The community treatment room

We include the community treatment room in our list of systems because it contains a lot of them, and the acupuncture is in some ways the least important. The seemingly simple process of a patient choosing her own chair and making herself comfortable before she meets with an acupuncturist is actually enormously significant to our business. It keeps the patient empowered and in control, which cannot be underestimated in the context of healthcare of any kind; it keeps the focus on the patient's experience and off the personality of the acupuncturist, by highlighting the patient's relationship to the treatment room itself.

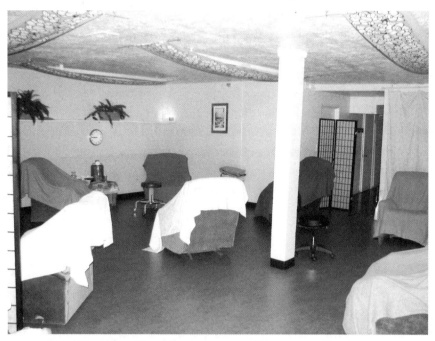

Working Class Acupuncture Treatment Room
(Groucho Room)

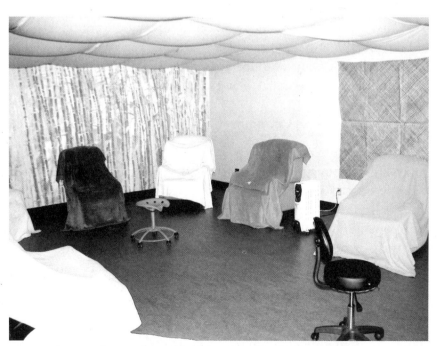

Working Class Acupuncture Treatment Room
(Chico Room)

That small period of time in which a patient prepares herself for treatment also has a positive impact on the clinical effectiveness of the acupuncture, because it represents a conscious process of focusing inward. When the patient walks into the treatment room after having paid and scheduled, she is leaving the rest of her world and her cares behind, at least as much as she can. She is taking time for herself, making her own sanctuary, actively participating in her healing. The fact that the treatment room is full of dozens of people doing this in sight of each other throughout the day makes the core of the clinic completely transparent. It reinforces the truth that what makes acupuncture work is what happens inside the patient; what the acupuncturist does merely facilitates it.

4. Simple paperwork

Because we do not bill insurance, our patient charts have only two purposes: to fulfill very basic legal requirements around record keeping, and to allow the acupuncturists to keep track of the patients' progress relative to the recipes they have been using. This makes our charting very simple and efficient, consisting primarily of the patient's concerns and the acupuncture points we used to address them. An acupuncturist can see up to 24 patients in a four hour shift and spend another half hour at the end filling in their charts.

Patients fill out short, focused health history forms on their first visit. They also sign an agreement to cancel or reschedule appointments with not less than 24 hours' notice, an informed consent to treatment, and an arbitration agreement from our professional liability insurance company.

5. Our systems are our marketing

We have learned that our potential patients cannot be educated about the benefits of acupuncture in the abstract. Citing favorable studies does not help; people mostly make appointments when they hear that acupuncture benefited someone whom they know personally. We estimate that 90% of our new patients come through word of mouth; most of the remaining 10% drive or walk by our building, see our five-foot red fist logo and get curious; a handful are referred by physicians and nurse practitioners, most of whom we have never met, who have heard from mutual patients that acupuncture is effective and that we are very serious about helping people get better. We have learned over the years that we need absolute consistency in our message, our operations, and our core philosophy. Our patients trust us with the health of their friends and family in part because we openly acknowledge the reality of class in America, we recognize its impact on healthcare, and we have organized every aspect of our business to explicitly address it.

Our operations are our marketing. Our sliding scale is our marketing because it allows patients at all different levels of income to receive enough acupuncture in order to get good results -- and when that happens, they talk about it. Our community treatment room is our marketing, because it allows people to see other people having a positive experience with acupuncture. About 20% of our new patients come in to the clinic for their first appointment with a friend or relative who is also a patient, and many of them, particularly married couples, continue the arrangement by scheduling their future appointments together. With regard to our operations, many of our patients are not just patients but "raving fans", to borrow Southwest Airlines' term; they love how we do things, and they show it by taking handfuls of our business cards to give away at work, by wearing our t-shirts and starting conversations about our clinic, and by coaxing their friends and relatives to try acupuncture. Because we have so many consistent systems, acupuncture is easy for our patients to describe and to promote. They know what will happen when they bring in their friends -- exactly what happened last time, exactly what they liked so much.

Why We Love Our Systems

We believe that simple, consistent systems are the key to acupuncture becoming widely embraced in America. Consistent, simple systems provide consistent, simple, positive experiences of acupuncture for large numbers of patients. Having systems, especially systems that empower patients, takes away any negative mystery associated with acupuncture while leaving all of the positive mystery intact. Consistent, simple systems create a container for the patient's healing process, in addition to making acupuncture safe to try and safe to recommend.

Sameness and ritual contribute to safety. For instance: all of the recliners in our treatment room are different, because they all come from different sources: patient donations, Craigslist, Goodwill, etc. We always joked about the fact that patients become attached to their favorite chairs, but we had no idea how serious the attachment was until recently. Last year, we had new floors installed at our clinic. This required moving all of our furniture, including every last second-hand recliner, out of the treatment room, and then moving all of it back in when the floors were done, which happened to occur about 9 pm. As our weary crew of acupuncturists was lugging the chairs back to their places, we looked up to find that several patients had appeared in our midst. They were just standing there, watching us. They are people who live in our neighborhood, they had a general idea of our project timeline, *and they had come to the clinic at 9 pm at night to make sure with their own eyes that we put their favorite chairs back in the right places, so that they could find them next time.*

The consistent, simple systems of our clinic combine to make acupuncture into a ritual for many of our patients. They love every part of it: filling out their checks in advance, giving them to the receptionist and chatting with her, making regular appointments, going back into the treatment room, finding their favorite chairs, snoozing for a peaceful hour or so. People love becoming acupuncture "regulars". We have several patients who have kept the same appointment times for five years running. Not everyone values acupuncture because it is exotic; many of our patients value it because it is routine, ordinary, and comforting.

We have noticed over the years that a lot of patients gravitate to acupuncture while they are going through transitions: having a baby, going back to school, getting a divorce, starting a new job, leaving an old one. For some reason acupuncture seems to help people navigate change. "That was a rough time and you guys really got me through it", as one patient said. But what did we do? Nothing in particular, except that we were always there, always the same -- and acupuncture not only reduces stress, it creates a feeling of stability.

This is a good time to revisit our earlier discussion about values and how they relate to class. People who have unlimited resources tend to value what is unusual, unique, and exotic; they can value those things, because they are not spending the majority of their energy on survival. When your resources are more limited, you are more careful with them; you have more need for predictability and consistency. You can't necessarily extend yourself toward the exotic and the unknown with impunity; you can't risk your time or your money or your energy, because you don't have a surplus of any of those things. Making acupuncture into a rarefied, unique experience does not necessarily make it appealing to working class and lower middle class people; it only makes acupuncture into something that looks like it might be more trouble than it's probably worth.

Many acupuncturists locate their practices in "integrative medicine centers" or "natural medicine centers" where acupuncture is one modality among many: naturopathy, reflexology, massage therapy, chiropractic, etc. The idea here seems to be to appeal to potential patients by offering them a wide range of "health care options". We initially met with a great deal of disbelief when we announced that our clinic was only going to offer acupuncture. We did this because we feel that offering acupuncture as only one of a long list of options makes getting acupuncture into something like going shopping, and it is designed to appeal to upper class and upper middle class patients. Having lots of choices is fun when you have lots of resources; when you don't have lots of resources and you're concerned about your health, having lots of choices is just stressful. Many of our patients are not shopping when they come in for acupuncture; they are in pain. Acupuncture is not a lifestyle accoutrement for working class patients: it's health care.

Having systems at all is an expression of lower middle class and working class values, because systems make acupuncture easier to share. The hallmark of the Zen-Spa Noodle and the White-Coat Noodle is their uniqueness. The Zen-Spa Noodle emphasizes the special status of the patient, while the White-Coat Noodle emphasizes the special status of the practitioner. Either way, it's very clear that complementary/alternative medicine is supposed to be something special, distinctive, not average or ordinary or mundane. Uniqueness works fine as a value in conjunction with upper class values like personal service, or upper middle class values like personal achievement. But if you insert uniqueness into this list: *family connections, frugality, hard work, stability, simplicity, ease, interdependence, creativity, resourcefulness, personal relationships, directness, and loyalty*, doesn't it stick out like a sore thumb? Uniqueness implies "all mine, only mine", and a lot of working class and lower middle class values are more social and more inclusive than that.

Not that working class and lower middle class people don't experience certain things as special, but uniqueness is just not a social goal in the same way as it is for upper class and upper middle class people. Recently, we had two patients call in for an appointment together. One of them, let's call him John, was a return patient, and he wanted to come in with his friend, Tanya, who was a new patient. Tanya was very nervous about getting acupuncture, but she had allowed John to persuade her because she had severely twisted her ankle, which made it impossible for her to do her job as a bartender. John and Tanya sat next to each other so that Tanya could watch John get needled first. "So", the acupuncturist said, pulling a stool up next to John, "I know why she's here, but what can I do for you?" He smiled widely. "Oh, nothing special. I'm just here for moral support."

This kind of interaction would not even be possible in a Zen-Spa clinic or a White-Coat clinic. For John, the only purpose of getting acupuncture that day was to share acupuncture with someone he cared about. He didn't need individual pampering and he didn't need an individual diagnosis. Acupuncture for him was not an individual experience at all, but a social occasion. Systems emphasize the aspects of acupuncture that people can hold in common.

Systems and Relationships

Acupuncturists who recoil from our business model often do so on the basis of what they describe as a need to have deep relationships with their patients, because they think that cultivating relationships is not compatible with a low-cost, high-volume clinic that has lots of systems. Acupuncturists in this camp have accused us of being "the Walmart of acupuncture" or "the McDonalds of acupuncture" or "an acupuncture factory". (Everyone catch the classism there? We sure hope so.) These acupuncturists also tend to assert that what makes acupuncture valuable to patients is not the acupuncture itself, but the lengthy face time with the practitioner. They believe that patients are coming to acupuncture specifically to get what they can't get from Western medicine: lots of personal, individualized attention. We think that there are some peculiar assumptions at work here, as well as a hefty dose of classism.

First, there is the equation of relationships with talking -- lengthy talking, punctuated by personal disclosures on the patient side and advice giving on the practitioner side. This equation works best for upper class or upper middle class women, but for lots of other people, especially men of all classes, it actually doesn't work so well. Many conventional acupuncture practices have a patient base that is 90% female; our clinic's base is closer to 60% women, 40% men. We maintain that we attract more male patients than conventional acupuncturists because we don't make them talk, we just give them acupuncture, which is what they came for.

We feel that we have very deep relationships with many of our patients, cultivated over months or years. We make an effort to be present with our patients when we see them, even if our conversations are brief. Being fully present in dozens or hundreds of ten minute increments adds up. We know what our patients look like when they're asleep; we know who snores and who needs three blankets. We meet our patients' loved ones, because we end up treating them too. This makes us think again about our teacher Yoshi's maxim that acupuncture requires you to develop your heart, your hands, and your head, in that order of importance. You can develop very deep relationships by using your heart and your hands; you don't need all the talking that depends on your head.

Second, there is a peculiar assumption that the most important relationship to the patient must be the relationship between the patient and the practitioner, defined by the patient being the center of attention for some defined, and paid-for, period of time. This seems to us like an interesting combination of classism and practitioner narcissism. *Doesn't everybody want more uninterrupted time with me?*

No, everybody doesn't. Many people are uncomfortable with intimacy that they have to pay for, at least outside of the upper class where personal assistants and life coaches and psychotherapists are common. Many of our patients wouldn't think of an hour of face time that comes with a price tag as a real relationship. Far more real to them are the relationships they have with their family members, their close friends, the people they share their lives with, and it's those relationships that the community acupuncture business model prioritizes. We are fairly confident that the vast majority of our patients would choose being able to get acupuncture with the people they love (because all of them can afford to get it, not to mention that they can actually get it in the same physical space at the same time) over having an hour alone with their acupuncturist, if that meant that the people they love couldn't afford to get acupuncture too. Similarly, a lot of our patients simply value our business model because they know that it means more people can get acupuncture; they would choose their community being able to have acupuncture over having an hour all by themselves alone with their acupuncturist.

Relationships that are mostly nonverbal, relationships with family members and friends, relationship with one's community -- all of these relationships are just as real and valid and significant to acupuncture as the relationship between a patient and a practitioner who are doing lots of talking. All of them are also perfectly compatible with our systems. Arguing against the community acupuncture model on the basis that it doesn't value relationships suggests a weirdly limited, classist and commercialized definition of "relationship".

Acupuncturists who have this limited definition of relationships within acupuncture do not realize that what they are limiting most is acupuncture itself. By making personal conversation the most important part of their treatment, they are making it virtually impossible for people to embrace acupuncture in large numbers. How can I recommend acupuncture to my boss or my friends or my mother-in-law if my experience of acupuncture is that it is more like a paid friendship with an acupuncturist? If it's that personal, how can anyone else really share it? Furthermore, many acupuncturists who emphasize "relationship" with their patients do so because they have no confidence in their acupuncture. And so they talk: about diet, about lifestyle, about emotions, about anything they can think of. What they talk about will often vary wildly from patient to patient, and of course, it varies even more wildly amongst acupuncturists. There is no real consistency possible when it comes to personal conversations.

What makes us most hopeful about the community acupuncture movement is that at least a hundred acupuncture clinics have adopted our systems. That means that a hundred or so clinics have dining rooms that function basically in the same way, which means that one of our patients in Portland can refer her mother to a community acupuncture clinic in Sarasota or Philadelphia or Austin or Minneapolis or St. Louis with some confidence. She will have a pretty good idea of what will happen when her mother walks into that clinic; it won't wholly depend on her mother's personality or the acupuncturist's personality or a combination of the two. A hundred clinics sharing consistent systems have the potential to normalize acupuncture in America for tens of thousands of patients. In other words, systems have the potential to build the foundation for a relationship between acupuncturists and patients on a large scale.

Money Systems

The original insight that led to the development of all of our business systems is, in hindsight, fairly embarrassing. It involves arithmetic. We made the transition from the conventional practice of seeing one patient at a time for a large amount of money to seeing many patients at a time for small amounts of money because we finally did some arithmetic. In 2002, the year we founded our clinic, the going rate for an acupuncture treatment was $60. Of course, nobody in our working class neighborhood could possibly afford that. One day we had the shattering realization that 60 divided by 4 equals 15. Instead of seeing one person an hour for $60, we could see 4 people an hour for $15, and make the same amount of money.

And of course, it would be a whole lot easier to find 4 people who could pay $15 for acupuncture on a regular basis than it would be to find someone who would pay $60 even once. And even if each person ended up spending $60 at our clinic, $60 for four visits would be much more likely to produce results than $60 for one visit. Since acupuncture needles cost about two cents per needle, the critical factor was not materials but time.

This is where the emphasis on silence came in. Running a community acupuncture clinic cannot be an exercise in financial martyrdom; in our case, martyrdom was not even a possibility, since we had no savings to speak of and needed to make a living, right quick. The clinic had to support itself and us.

It rapidly became clear to us that if we were going to provide acupuncture to lots of people in our neighborhood, we could only provide acupuncture. We couldn't provide lots of talking, or lots of massage, or lots of the other time intensive things that other acupuncturists provide, or the arithmetic would no longer work out. If you are going to treat lots of people for little money, you have to treat them quickly, efficiently, and mostly silently.

Of course, what we found when we embraced these limitations was essentially an entirely new universe of acupuncture and of business. We had no idea how freeing it would be to rely upon acupuncture alone to help people feel better, or what a pleasure it would be to watch a room full of people sleeping with needles. We did not realize that we had been lonely in our previous conventional acupuncture practices until we discovered community acupuncture, and were no longer lonely.

Besides the desire to make acupuncture accessible to more people, this is a major reason we began reaching out to other acupuncturists: we knew that lots of them were lonely. As we watched other acupuncturists experiment with aspects of our model, we learned a few more things about the combination of community and systems. A lot of acupuncturists hoped to take some aspects of our model and keep aspects of the conventional acupuncture model: either insurance billing, or treating some patients privately, or trying to come up with other ways to treat people for less money without having everyone using a sliding scale. What we found with all of these attempted combinations is that they screw up our beloved systems.

Imagine a restaurant where every table in the dining room had a different menu; where some customers paid for their food when they ate but others had someone else pay for them, possibly months afterwards; where some customers could negotiate the price of their food but others couldn't; where some customers got discounts on their food because they were students or temporarily unemployed, but had to prove it; where the rules were completely different for different people. Do you think hungry people would find this complexity stimulating and fascinating? Or would they find it weird and confusing, because they just wanted to eat, and so they would avoid this restaurant like the plague?

Insurance billing is like some customers getting some other business to pay for their food, months after they eat it. Insurance does not work with the community acupuncture model because it has nothing to do with community. Insurance is someone else's system -- and that someone is a big, for-profit corporation. Insurance makes autonomy impossible. It also makes consistency impossible, since different insurance companies have different rules and different policies, which is like every table in the restaurant having a different menu.

Some acupuncturists believe that you can make acupuncture accessible to people of ordinary incomes by charging high market rates for acupuncture, but by offering lots of different discounts: for students, for retired people, for anyone who seems to them to deserve it. Discounts are not a system; they are an attempt to make exceptions to a system that isn't working. This is like a restaurant where some people can negotiate the price of their food, and others can't.

Some acupuncturists also hope to make the finances of their clinic viable by charging some patients more money for treatments in private cubicles in order to fund low cost community acupuncture for everybody else. Like discounts, this is not a system, but an attempt to find ways around a system that already isn't working. How do you explain this arrangement to a prospective customer in a way that doesn't identify the community treatments as inherently inferior? Why would the same service cost so much more? Would you want to go to a restaurant where you knew you would be treated better if only you had more money? Would you feel welcome there?

Inconsistent, overly individualized financial systems are just as much of a problem as inconsistent, overly individualized clinical systems for acupuncture: they make people not want to try it because they're hard to understand. If we want people to embrace acupuncture in large numbers, how they pay for acupuncture can't be complex or confusing. It has to be simple and consistent.

Since the late 1970s, long before Harry Potter came along, the acupuncture profession in America has been attracting people (mostly white people) who wanted to think of themselves as wizards. Acupuncture is magical, and that holds a certain appeal to the ego: if I know how to do acupuncture, I must be a magician, powerful and mysterious because I possess this ancient, arcane knowledge. The acupuncturist-as-wizard self-image leads to an unhealthy emphasis, at all levels of acupuncture practice, on the individual rather than on systems. The point of being a wizard is being a really special individual; if you're a wizard you don't have to be consistent, and you certainly don't need systems. You can do whatever you want, and unfortunately, that is the reason that a lot of people decided to become acupuncturists, so that they could be magical and whimsical and inscrutable and absolutely unaccountable.

Just because acupuncturists are in love with their own uniqueness does not mean that patients are, however. Business practices that are esoteric and unfathomable are not, in fact, charming; complexity repels rather than attracts most people. Acupuncturists would be much better off as a profession if we collectively got over ourselves and decided to be cooks rather than wizards.

Social Business, Money, and Self Respect

The community acupuncture business model basically fits the definition of a "social business" as defined by Nobel Peace Prize winner Dr. Muhammad Yunus in his book, Creating A World Without Poverty. A social business is designed to create social benefits rather than profits. It is not the same as a nonprofit corporation, however, because a nonprofit typically depends on money in the form of grants or donations that was originally made elsewhere; a social business makes its own money. A social business is also not the same as a socially responsible business, because a socially responsible business takes a percentage of its profits and gives them to other, separate nonprofits. A social business does not necessarily make any profit above what it needs to operate; its goal is simply to exist.[1]

A community acupuncture clinic is designed to create the twin social benefits of inexpensive acupuncture for everyone and stable, living wage jobs for acupuncturists. Between trying to keep the bottom end of the sliding scale low enough to be affordable to working class people and trying to keep the wages of the acupuncturists high enough to live on, there is nothing left over for profits. (So if anyone hoping to make a quick buck off of the revolution actually waded this far through the book, you can stop reading now. No profits, quick or otherwise.) Wages without profits are fine with us, in part because we feel genuinely queasy about the idea of making a profit while practicing healthcare. We know that people may find us quaint for saying so, but we believe that there is a moral problem with making money off of human suffering. We need to be compensated for taking care of people, certainly, because it takes up our time and energy and prevents us from earning a living any other way -- but being compensated with a paycheck is different than setting up our business so that sick people pay more than they absolutely have to for care in order for us to accumulate money without working for it. Some acupuncturists whom we otherwise respect keep promoting the idea that everyone should charge their patients lots of money so that acupuncturists can become rich and give money away to charities who will then do good works; we find this a very weird and convoluted kind of altruism. If you want to do good, why not just do it yourself? With people you know? Right now, instead of waiting to accumulate enough money to give away to someone else to do it?

One of the most revolutionary aspects of the community acupuncture movement is the idea, which we got from Dr. Yunus, that capitalism can be used for something other than accumulating money. *That the point of owning a business is not to make money, it's to make something happen.* We have found that both owning a social business and working in one makes a lot of things happen for us. Not just affordable acupuncture and stable acupuncture jobs, but some really great internal things as well.

Self-respect is one great internal thing that happens. For many people, everything having to do with money, including business, is infused with fear, guilt, hopelessness, powerlessness and scarcity. All of that changes – because it has to change – when you create your own livelihood by doing something that you believe in wholeheartedly. Owning your own business, especially when it is a social business, is not unlike owning your own universe. In our universe, all of the people in our neighborhood can afford acupuncture. We made it so. As a result, we believe in ourselves and we respect ourselves.

Demystification of capitalism also happens, and it is another great thing. It would be an even greater thing if it happened more often. The specter of capitalism has way more power than it deserves in the lives of a lot of people who think of themselves as good, or spiritual, or progressive. There is the feeling that only bad people really understand money and business, and they use their money and their businesses for their bad, exploitative ends. Good people may interact with money and business only as necessary evils, but they are not supposed to actually like or understand them. If you are a good person, you are a victim of capitalism, and if you're a victim of capitalism, you must be a good person. We have come to think of these beliefs as the way that good people abdicate responsibility for the world. Capitalism has shaped much of the world, and if you refuse to understand it, you can't participate in reshaping those parts of the world. You can make capitalism do whatever you want it to do, but not if you don't know how it works.

Business, capitalist business, is not particularly difficult to understand. It involves arithmetic, and patience, and attention, but it isn't rocket science. We agree wholeheartedly with Dr. Yunus that anyone can be a business owner; entrepreneurship is a basic human capacity.[2] If good people refuse to learn about business because they don't want to get their hands dirty, of course bad people will dominate business and use it for bad ends. It's not that business is unfathomable and inherently sinister, or that bad people are cunning and powerful, it's just that a lot of good people are lazy. Acupuncturists who blame the insurance companies for people not being able to get acupuncture are being lazy; they are allowing someone else to decide how the business of acupuncture happens.

We are not suggesting that running any business, including a social business, is easy. It's not easy – but it is potentially quite simple. Anyone who wants to do it badly enough can learn. Taking the time and the trouble to learn will also create self-respect. We should warn everyone that you might have to give up some things to successfully run a business, though. You have to give up chaos and drama in your personal life. You have to give up being passive. You have to give up the hope that somebody or something else is going to rescue you – and yes, we include the dream of single payer healthcare in America. If you are an acupuncturist, the government is not going to rescue you from having to be in business by establishing single payer healthcare that pays for unlimited amounts of acupuncture for everyone. Sorry. In short, if you want to run a business – instead of leaving business to the bad people and then complaining – you need to grow up and take responsibility for yourself. <u>In Creating a World Without Poverty</u>, Dr. Yunus describes beggars in Bangladesh taking out microcredit loans in order to become door-to-door peddlers, otherwise known as "self sufficient small business owners".[3] Think about that – if beggars in Bangladesh are willing to learn how to run a business, what exactly is YOUR excuse?

The ultimate and true reward for running a social business is that you get to live out your values, and your values are people and relationships rather than money and status. The community acupuncture business model is based on the belief that people are valuable, specifically people who are often not treated as valuable. In its own way, this is as unfamiliar in America as acupuncture itself.

The social business model seems to us to be especially suited to acupuncture, because acupuncture is inherently so simple and so inexpensive. It needs so little to work so well. Just as acupuncture does not fit into the Western medical paradigm, neither does it fit into the typical American business paradigm. It's hard to squeeze profits out of acupuncture, but it's easy to use acupuncture for the benefit of many people. Acupuncture works best when it is allowed to be its humble, useful, radically unselfish self.

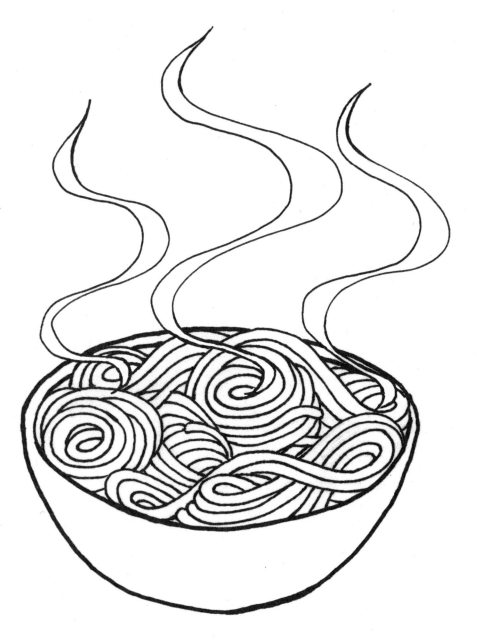

Part Four: Reflections on the Kitchen and the Dining Room, from Several Different Angles

As part of our participation in the Community Acupuncture Network, we started a blog that we named "Prick, Prod, and Provoke", which was designed to get people, especially acupuncturists, thinking about issues related to community acupuncture. Here are some of the blog posts written by Working Class Acupuncture employees, which we think provide valuable perspectives on cooking, serving, and understanding noodles.

What's the Point of the Community Acupuncture Business Model? By Skip

Short Answer:

Within the context of economic reality, to allow acupuncturists to both make a living and develop themselves as practitioners, while being allowed to be acupuncturists as opposed to having to be all sorts of other things.

Long Answer:

Who are we?

We're acupuncturists. Not medical doctors, not psychotherapists, not estheticians, not junior shamans or chiropractors or psychics.

What are we trying to do?

Make a living by doing acupuncture. Provide for us and for our loved ones. We want to make money by doing something we find interesting.

How do we make a living by doing acupuncture?

By seeing enough clients at a given rate per client to cover expenses. Hopefully we make more money than is needed to just break even.

In a real way this is just like a salesman who is paid by commission and who must make quota every month to stay employed. Most acupuncturists are self-employed but we have the same very real high pressure need to make quota (which in our case means living expenses).

Normally an acupuncturist rents office space either by themselves or in collaboration with other health care practitioners. This space typically has one or two rooms with a massage table in each plus a reception/waiting area. Prices per client typically range between $50-$250 per session. The average in Portland is about $75. For the purposes of this book we use $60 per treatment as the going rate. Now come the problems.

Defining the Market

The first problem is that you are confining yourself to a niche market. In other words most people can't afford you. To better understand this, look at paying $60 or more per treatment from the patient's point of view. Take a look at some census data, specifically household income data from 2005:

Household Income	% of Total Households
Less than $10,000	8.7%
$10,000 to $14,999	6.2%
$25,000 to $24,999	12.0%
$25,000 to $34,999	11.5%
$35,000 to $49,999	15.1%
$50,000 to $74,999	18.9%
$75,000 to $99,999	11.4%
$100,000 to $149,999	10.1%
$150,000 to $199,999	3.2%
$200,000 or more	3.0%
Median Income	$46,242
Mean Income	$62,556

[factfinder.census.gov]

So in looking at this table I'll first separate out the households in the lowest 14.9%, those households with incomes lower than 15K. Most of these folks -- but not all -- are below the US official poverty level. (The reason I say "most" is that the definition of a household varies from a single person living alone to a family of 5, 6, 7 whatever.) It is these folks that public health initiatives focus on.

Next I will take out the highest 6.2%- those households with incomes above 150K. This includes every rich person and much of the upper middle class. It is our contention that the acupuncture industry primarily targets this group. These folks do not have to think much at all about income and cash flow when they decide to get an acupuncture treatment. (Well, actually, that's not completely fair as Lisa has a college professor patient whose husband's an MD -- but her mom has Alzheimer's, her sister has cancer, she has several kids and ... she likes paying our rates and won't go to a typical practice that charges $75 . People's real lives are often a lot more complicated than those income charts reflect.)

That leaves those households with incomes above 15K and below 150K; the incomes that we put in boldface in the above table. **79% of all US households**. Most of these households need to check their cash flow before spending $60, 75, 100, 150 or more (if they are going more than once a week which is usually the smart thing to do when getting acupuncture). It's these **79% of all households** that have to balance where their money goes.

Now it stands to reason if these **79%** need to look at their bank balance then the more often they need to go, the less likely they will finish a full course of treatment as each session takes another bite out of their income. As acupuncturists we see this problem all the time. Patients say things like they can only come once or twice a month or they call up after hours and cancel their next appointment or they say they can't afford the herbs that are an additional cost or they say they just aren't getting any results. These things happen and many acupuncturists have a funny way of rationalizing the loss of what is a decent percentage of their income. They say, "Well if they were really committed to their health they wouldn't stop seeing me."

To us that's a prime instance of not seeing the forest for the trees, because these acupuncturists are not taking into consideration what their patients are thinking about, what their worries are and what their responsibilities are. These acupuncturists are thinking that the patient's decision to discontinue treatment is ultimately about their relationship with acupuncture or the acupuncturist, rather than about everything else in the patient's life, that there's a failure to prioritize rather than a sober evaluation of what's possible with limited resources. Too often acupuncturists think that when someone walks through their door that they should become a top priority in that person's life.

That's never the case though. The fact is that people go through life in pain: physical pain, emotional pain, mental pain, spiritual pain. It's the human condition. It should go without saying then that everyone is balancing how to deal with that pain while they take care of their responsibilities to the other people in their lives. The decision to see an acupuncturist is never a completely isolated decision. It's always weighed against everything else in their lives. For **79% of all households** their other concerns are always at least almost as important as going to an acupuncturist. Unless the acupuncturist realizes this and takes into consideration the patient's whole life in setting prices and treatments strategies than they are choosing to disregard many of the primary concerns of the great majority of Americans, and so they relegate themselves to a narrow niche market. In fact that's what acupuncture is in America: a niche product. This wonderful medicine has precious little impact on America's health; much less than chiropractors, not even in the same league as allopathic medicine.

I Can't Get No Satisficaction

Here's another way to talk about this problem. Have you ever heard of the word satisficing? It's a word coined by Herb Simon who won a Nobel prize in Economics for it. He was most interested in how people make decisions.

Here's what Wikipedia says about satisficing:

> In economics, satisficing is a behavior which attempts to achieve at least some minimum level of a particular variable, but which does not necessarily maximize its value ... The word satisfice was coined by Herbert Simon. **Simon pointed out that human beings lack the cognitive resources to maximize: we usually do not know the relevant probabilities of outcomes, we can rarely evaluate all outcomes with sufficient precision, and our memories are weak and unreliable.**
> [en.wikipedia.org]

So in thinking of getting treated with acupuncture, these **79% of all US households** satisfice. They try to juggle all the demands in their lives to the best of their abilities. That includes their health and the health of their families. Basically they are just trying to get by in the best way that they know. If their health is good enough they are less likely to start or continue treatment, and they are less likely to start or continue treatment is the treatment is expensive. If they start or continue treatment they have to either REALLY like the treatment and/or the treatment is cheap enough that it doesn't enter into their satisficing process enough to put up red flags.

Almost everyone in this middle **79% of all US households** don't have much of an understanding of acupuncture. That's true even if they've been needled several times. It's a healing modality they didn't grow up with as it's not yet a part of the warp and woof of our society. Yin and yang etc. are foreign concepts. I'm not saying we must discard those concepts like some acupuncturists say. Far from it: I love those concepts. But if we are to get these **79% of all US households** to darken our doors we must make it easy for them to say yes. Among other things that includes removing price as much as possible from the satisficing being done by our customers.

Practice Building

To make a living at $60 a treatment, an acupuncturist needs to see at least 15 clients per week- and that's only if you are living modestly and providing only for yourself since that gets you only $900 for that week and that's before taxes and expenses. A major problem stands out in this scenario:

Attracting a minimum of 15 clients per week (preferably more).

Sustaining a practice of attracting at least 15 clients per week, every week, is no easy task. First there is the problem of building up to that level, something that many new acupuncturists never achieve. Acupuncturists have tried all sorts of advertising to attract new clients and what's been found is that there is no advertising that supplies a steady stream of clients. The only thing that works is word of mouth but to do that you need satisfied clients talking you up to their friends and acquaintances.

A common way around this starting-a-new-practice dilemma is by temporarily reducing your fees- even giving free treatments. But the problem there is that eventually you will need to start charging full price to stay open and often those clients who got the cut rate stop coming at full price and/or they don't recommend you at full price.

But say you do attract some full price paying clients. Here's where the cycle gets vicious. Most conditions that clients have require repeated treatments because the symptoms the clients are complaining about are related to a larger syndrome that the acupuncturist must address to bring relief. (This is especially true for new acupuncturists who might not have the ability to bring about at least some relief on the first treatment.) But at $60 a treatment most clients are shy at investing potentially hundreds and thousands of dollars over a period of time in an acupuncturist to get better when they have no guarantee that they will indeed get better.

In other words, acupuncture is a long-term strategy but most patients are only willing to put in short-term money to get satisfaction: they just don't feel they can afford a full course of treatment.

What is written above tends to be true for chronic problems, but if the injury is acute, there are also problems as it's best to see the client more than once per week. However most clients will balk at paying $120/week or more (maybe much more) for pain relief.

Ah, but what about insurance? Aren't people more likely to see an acupuncturist if they are insured? The answer is yes, but...

First of all, most people don't have insurance that covers acupuncture, so right off the bat you are eliminating way more than 70% of the population from seeing you. Second, if you have a client that is covered, you run into several problems in getting that money. The insurance company will probably limit the number of treatments the client can get and if they aren't "cured" at the end of those sessions then it's likely that your client will stop seeing you -- and won't be satisfied (no chance of word of mouth referrals).

Then there's the reimbursing problem. If you bill the insurance company it can take weeks to get reimbursed, messing with your cash flow. Various snafus happen causing the insurer to delay payment to you. (And why should they be prompt anyway? You're not their client.) If you have several clients that you are billing insurance companies for, the amount of paperwork involved seriously cuts into your time and you start to work several more hours per week for which you are not getting paid at all. OR you can hire a billing specialist. ("One of the fastest growing professions in America!" says my local technical college on TV.) Of course by doing so you create more overhead putting pressure on you to do one or both of the following: raise your rates and/or see more clients per week.

Can you see the vicious cycle here: raising your rates cuts down on the number of people who can afford you which directly affects your ability to attract new clients?

You might think that if you can get enough clients then you wouldn't have to care about your noninsured population, but that supposes that in the long run that more and more people will be getting acupuncture insurance. Given that the health insurance business is in a retracting mode -- fewer people have any kind of insurance these days -- it seems far-fetched that more folks will get acupuncture insurance.

But let's say that you are able to get 15 or more clients a week. But you are not out of the woods yet. Now comes the problem of what you doing all this work for anyway.

Keeping Life Interesting

We all became acupuncturists because at some level we find the medicine fascinating. Furthermore, a large proportion of us changed careers to become acupuncturists, so we are comparing it to what we have experienced before. But a subtle problem insidiously creeps up on us: if we are not careful, the art will become boring while at the same time we are tense trying to make ends meet. Let's see how this happens:

It takes experience to become a really good acupuncturist. All else being equal, clients are more likely to see a more experienced acupuncturist. You need to see lots of clients to get that experience and you need to see them over many, many treatments, preferably over years, to really improve yourself.

Getting good in the profession doesn't mean merely paying your license fees for a bunch of years. It also doesn't mean attending a lot of continuing education CEU seminars. It means figuring out what works for you, developing your own style. This is a never-ending process really. Acupuncturists who've been practicing 30 years keep learning just as much as a brand new practitioner. But the problem for a practitioner is that in order to develop oneself, one must take risks with one's clients. Try out new techniques and new theories. In other words take the risk that your clients may not like how you treated them yesterday as much as they liked their treatment last week. They may not get any relief with your latest experiment and/or they may have found it unpleasant even if they got relief. If this happens you risk losing that patient.

An example of this type of risk is the transition that many practitioners have made from using local points for pain to using distal points (such as Dr. Tan's Balance method). Some patients might initially be skeptical. "How can points in my hand treat my back pain?" Over time, however, patients may find that the distal treatments are actually more effective - but getting to that point may require risking patients' displeasure or disbelief.

If you want to get better you *have* to take those risks. But if you are just making ends meet your impulse is to get conservative, to make the client have as enjoyable a treatment as possible - whether or not it's what that client needs -- so they are more likely to come back. After all if you lose one of your 15 clients in a week, you lose 6.67% of your income for at least that week- a big loss if you think about it.

It would be best if you saw enough clients a week that you didn't worry unduly about your clients' preferences and felt free to do what you saw needed to be done to get them to a higher level of health. By charging $60 (or higher) a treatment your client base and potential populations is likely to be limited so you stay with the tried and true- which may not be what's most effective. Being a good practitioner sometimes means telling patients something they don't want to hear, or pursuing a path of treatment they wouldn't choose themselves. You sometimes have to choose between making someone happy with you for an hour and helping them get well and stay well.

If conservative treatments become your pattern out of fear, if you are basically doing the same thing week after week, year after year, then your practice becomes an auto assembly line - uninspired and ineffective - making it harder and harder to attract new clients and even more important boring to you. People like some change in their lives and acupuncturists are no exception.

Looking at Units

We've just discussed the vicious cycle of $60 treatments coupled with 15-20 treatments per week. Briefly, the problems with this model are:

1. People don't like spending the amount of money needed for enough treatments to really address the root of their problems, so

2. It's hard for the practitioner to really develop his art.

So how do you get out of this cycle? Simple: change your price cycle so clients are both more likely to try acupuncture (thus increasing the number of clients) and they are more likely to stick with it (increasing both client satisfaction and practitioner knowledge). In other words: **lower your prices**.

Say you lowered your fee from $60 to $30 a treatment. You would then need twice as many clients to make the same amount of money. But why would practitioners want to do this? To develop their art (and thus themselves). Again, in order to become a better practitioner one needs to treat a lot of people. Thousands, really. Tens of thousands of treatments. Ideally you should be spending all of your working hours (up to 30 hours a week) treating people. But if you only see 15 people a week you aren't seeing nearly enough clients to get to be any good and you have a whole lot of dead time on your hands- time that you should be treating people if only they would pay your rate.

Why not double the number of clients to 30? How about 45? 50? 60? Now we're talking! You'd be seeing a much more diverse population (a broader range of syndromes and conditions) plus (and this is important) you'd be free to try out new techniques because if a client or two didn't like your treatments it would barely affect your cash flow. The truly creative acupuncturist in you would be released and trying new things is the only way you get good.

Take a look at this table:

Client Treatments			
Per week	Per 4 weeks	Per 50 week/year	Per decade
15	60	750	7,500
30	120	1500	15,000
45	180	2250	22,500
60	240	3000	30,000
75	300	3750	37,500
100	400	5000	50,000

Practically by definition the busier the practitioner the faster they develop and the happier they are, because as each particular treatment means less in terms of money earned, the more likely it becomes that the practitioner will feel free to be creative. And creativity is fun. And that's the point.

Just the Acupuncture Part
By John

One of the acupuncturists who works in our clinic, John Vella, recently summed up how a community acupuncturist approaches treating a lot of patients in small increments of time. He said, " I realize that I'm not responsible for my patient's whole entire life -- I'm just responsible for the acupuncture part."

This means that in interacting with patients, a community acupuncturist only needs to get enough information in order to do a good job with the acupuncture part. You don't need to know everything, you just need to know enough to do a good treatment.

Tales from the Trenches: My Paradigm Shift from TCM to Community Acupuncture
by Moses

Hi, my name is Moses and I work with Lisa and Skip in the Working Class Acupuncture clinic here in Portland, Oregon. As an acupuncturist who works in the WCA clinic, I thought some of you might be interested in my personal paradigm shift from traditional Chinese medicine (TCM) style practice to community acupuncture (CA).

For me, moving from TCM into CA has been a process of understanding subtle differences between these two styles. During my work with WCA I've had to reexamine my understanding of what TCM has to offer. I've also had to consider that less patient-practitioner interaction may be a benefit, which was at odds with my standard TCM training. Finally, I have witnessed over and over again the healing aspects of group treatments, where patients are brought together in silence to heal, which is an experience unique to CA.

Before I explain my paradigm shift, though, first let me tell you about how I became connected to CA style acupuncture. I met Lisa while she was selling her original Little Red Book at an Oregon Acupuncture Association conference. As a recent graduate from acupuncture school, I was collecting information about how to set up a practice and the community approach was very interesting. After reading the Little Red Book, I made an appointment at Lisa's clinic to experience the community atmosphere first hand. The clinic reminded me of a home more than an office, with its natural warmth and casual atmosphere. I noticed that I felt at ease there and was quite excited to try acupuncture in a recliner. Coming from a TCM practice background, I wasn't yet aware that you could use distal points primarily, but found it very effective and relaxing.

In June 2005 I began a one-year mentorship at WCA and at the end of the mentorship began working as a licensed acupuncturist at the clinic. As an acupuncturist I strive to offer my patients the best that acupuncture and oriental medicine (AOM) has to offer. The common interpretation of the best of AOM is something I have been challenged to redefine since working with the WCA team and this is where my paradigm shift comes in.

I learned in acupuncture school that the best way to provide acupuncture and oriental medicine care, and to make a good living while doing so, was to offer as many high quality healing therapies as possible to whoever can pay for your services. The "whoever can pay for your services" line translated to me as: charge current market rates for acupuncture and see a clientele that you may not naturally connect with outside of acupuncture practice. I am a skateboarder from a working class family in rural BC, Canada. My inspiration to study acupuncture came from my own experience of receiving effective pain relief through acupuncture. I used acupuncture and qigong exercise to heal from intense joint pains, developed through labor work and skateboarding, and after my acupuncture experience I wanted to offer this same healing potential to everyone in my community. The idea of charging my patients more than I could reasonably afford always made me feel uneasy. Through my years of training, this dilemma stayed in the back of my mind as something to resolve some day when I was practicing. I thought to myself, "Once I'm practicing, I'll have this ethical piece figured out. Just hang in there and it will be addressed before I graduate." The issues of classism and ease of access to acupuncture care were never acknowledged during my four years in acupuncture school. The CA business model felt like a sort of cavalry that arrived just in time for me to practice acupuncture with a clear conscience. However, I have only recently understood what I feel are the core differences between standard TCM and CA.

For most of my mentorship and professional practice at the WCA clinic I was treating people using a trimmed down TCM acupuncture style. In the TCM treatment approach patients are asked to think about many details of their health history which tends to result in mild anxiety instead of relaxation. Lisa's new book, The Remedy, has helped me to shift my thinking about what professional acupuncture is for, and how the delivery of this medicine can better fit the realities of working class patients.

I find that CA style intake focuses only on essential data for treatment, and makes treating the patient effectively and efficiently the primary goal. The benefit of this efficient treatment style is a more calming and comfortable experience for patients. Patients that are calm and comfortable feel safe and tend to go within, where the healing takes place, more deeply. With CA I notice that over the course of treatment as tensions fade in my patients they become more acutely aware of their overall health condition. This internal awareness seems to develop as the treatments progress and I notice they incrementally make more health benefiting decisions in their lives. I feel that this awareness process shows that the most dramatic personal changes happen when patients have the quiet and stillness to change on their own terms. Health recommendations and suggestions are always useful when appropriate, though it seems to me that most patients need a certain amount of treatment before they are ready to make any new personal health decisions. This is an example of how I find that there is less need for talk and more time for the treatment experience in the CA model than in the TCM approach.

Another unique benefit of the CA model is the group treatment setting. I became particularly aware of this advantage recently while treating a new patient. This patient told me during the intake that her friends tell her that she needs to calm down and that she is "too high strung" for her own good. I noticed that this patient had a difficult time with silence. She was clearly used to living with a high level of anxiety, and expected me to counsel her about it like others had done for her in the past. Recognizing that what this patient really needed was to calm down and allow her body-mind to relax, I guided her into the treatment room as soon as the essential intake discussion was complete. Shared silence carries a side benefit of respecting other peoples' healing experience by talking quietly or not at all. As soon as this patient entered the community acupuncture room her voice went low, and once the needles were in she was fast asleep in just a few moments. I feel her experience is worth relating as an example of how the CA clinic format encourages even our most anxious patients to calm down naturally.

Transitioning from TCM style patient interaction into CA has been an ongoing process of shifting subtle ways that I interact with my patients. Working with the WCA team has helped me reexamine what TCM has to offer and which parts of it fit in the CA model. Consciously encouraging less patient/ practitioner verbal interaction is a unique experience and benefit to the healing process in CA. Group treatments offer a setting that is calming by itself. It is always a pleasure to bring people into a room full of healing energy. Less talk, more stillness. It's been a good lesson for me. I hope this is helpful to anyone considering the shift from TCM style interaction, toward a more efficient and very effective CA style approach.

A Glimpse of Community Acupuncture in Action

Here is a glimpse of what a typical acupuncture shift is like at the Working Class Acupuncture clinic.

It's Tuesday morning at 8:00 AM and I have just arrived at the clinic. My shift is from 8:30 to 12:30 and I hope to see around twenty patients this morning. There are 18 people scheduled in ten minute increments and that leaves room for about 4 more call-ins (new patients get two appointment spaces and I have two new patients today).

Sandy arrived a few minutes ago and put out the front door mat and brought last evenings cups into the kitchen. While she unloads the clean cups for the day and re-loads the dishwasher I walk through the clinic and check that all lights, heaters, and fountains are turned on. Once the gas ceiling heater is humming above me I make the rounds and visit each recliner and table to fluff the fleece cover and change out those that need to be changed.

It is now 8:10, I have finished preparing the treatment room and am off to look through my charts for the day. Sandy has photocopied my schedule and put it on my desk and I feel a sense of appreciation to all of our receptionists for all that they do to make my acupuncture work easier. I highlight the new patients on my schedule and then fold it so it fits neatly in my back pocket. With my treatment schedule in my pocket I start to skim through all of my patient charts for the day, noting patients that I am familiar with and patients I will be meeting for the first time. I place my stack of charts on my desk and file through the top layer, taking a moment to memorize the names and chief concerns of the first five patients of the morning.

As I do this the copper bell tied to the front door chimes and I hear the voice of my first patient, who takes a seat at the front desk and begins chatting with Sandy. By 8:25 the first patient has paid and gone back into the treatment room to settle into a reclining chair. I am ready to begin treatments and take a moment to stretch while I let my first patient get settled. As I enter the treatment room I notice that the overhead heater has been on high long enough and I turned it down to keep the treatment room at a comfortable temperature.

I then roll a stool over to my patient's chair, open a new package of needles, and rub my hands with sanitizer gel. I say hello to my patient, and ask how her hip is doing today. She replies that the pain is around five out of ten (1 is low intensity and 10 is high intensity) but that the location is more generally in the low back since last treatment four days ago and she feels less shooting pain in the hip and down the back of the leg now. I nod and say that I am pleased with the progress thus far. I check her wrist and neck pulses to determine the Jingei ratio and I come up with 2:1, arm, indicating small intestine as the main channel to focus on. Since her pain has moved from specifically sciatic type pain to more generalized low back pain I revise the treatment from last session by a few points and yet maintain a strong focus on treating the Taiyang channels and specifically the low back area.

As I place the needles she inquires about treatment frequency and I tell her that two times per week is still recommended right now since her pain level is over five out of ten. I remark that once the pain has subjectively dropped to a four out of ten for a whole week I would recommend her shifting to one treatment per week. She says that sounds reasonable and as I place the last needle I wish her a good rest. The heat is at a comfortable level now and I move on to the next patient.

I notice two more patients have entered the room and have started to settle into their recliners. As I think back to my list I note that one is the patient I haven't met yet but who has been regularly seeing another acupuncturist at the clinic and the other across the room is someone I know. Everyone is slightly early this morning and I like that. I greet the next patient by introducing myself and making sure to note his name to be sure it is the patient on my list. I have already read through his chart and ask him what he would like to focus on today. He says that his headaches are back and he has a mild one right now, but his left ankle is feeling much better, so could we do a little bit of both. This patient has lifelong migraine headaches on the right side behind his eye. After weekly treatments for three months the headaches have gone from daily to about once per week if at all, and the intensity of pain has gone from around six to eight out of ten consistently to around two to four out of ten if they come up at all. This patient is very easygoing and I find a quick connection and trust developing as I place the needles. I say nice to meet you and ask him if he wants a blanket before moving to my third patient of the day.

My third patient is a regular that comes in to counter the exhaustion that comes with radiation therapy. She has been working through cancer and the treatment effects are promising, yet each bout of radiation leaves her feeling drained and vulnerable to colds. Today she has a productive cough, clear and thin sputum, and is very tired. She finds that acupuncture helps her make it through each week. She comes twice a week and it is clear that the acupuncture is keeping her going. I know this patient well and as we exchange greetings she is already settling into a restful state. I cover my third patient with a blanket even though the room is warm. Her body needs all the external warmth it can get right now. Once the first three patients are relaxing peacefully, I glance around the room taking in all that is going on. Everyone is resting comfortably so I start toward the charting room in the front of the clinic. I notice my fourth patient is calmly sipping tea and my fifth has just walked through the front entry, sounding the chime of our door bell. I greet them both, glance at the schedule on the front desk and make my way to the back room to chart.

As I think through my first treatment of the morning I jot down "low back pain" under subjective, "2:1, arm channel and wiry" under objective, "focus on small intestine channel" under assessment, and under plan I write: "repeat treatment 11/03/07", and note the 3 points that were added today and the 4 points that were left out based on the changing location of the pain. For my second patient I put "mild right sided headache behind eye and ankle pain improving, still lateral GB 40 area (Shaoyang)". Under objective I note "1.5:1, leg channel and slightly rapid pulse". Assessment is "focus on the gall bladder channel". For the treatment plan I draw a cross on the page and note the acupoint numbers under each of the four quadrants of the body. At the end of each charted entry I draw a line to the edge of the page and sign my name. It has been about five minutes since my fifth patient came in the door so instead of looking at my third chart I memorize the names and chief complaints of my next 5 patients and leave the charting room to treat my fourth and fifth patients of the day.

As I make my way through the work day in the clinic I develop a rhythm to how I think and move. I am always keeping an eye on the treatment room as a whole while moving from patient to patient. When I notice one of my patients has started to stir from their slumber I prioritize unpinning before starting my next treatment.

Tending to a room full of patients becomes an opportunity to learn how to stay in a flow state while simultaneously developing technical and interpersonal skills as an acupuncturist. When six to ten patients are resting in treatment at one time it creates a palpable restful energy, and I use this environmental influence to stay relaxed and move smoothly through the treatment processes. Clinically speaking, community acupuncture is a mix of making specific health assessments quickly coupled with observing the group of patients as a whole. My day is made up of a series of small moments that when looked at in sequence seem very busy, yet in real time each moment is given careful attention.

I make an effort to talk as little as possible in the treatment room, I remember Lisa referring to this as an economy of dialogue, where you concisely discuss the main points of health issues with your patients on follow up visits. I also make an effort to finish with my current patient within about five minutes when I see that another patient is waiting for me. This awareness of timing maintains the flow, and encourages a smooth pace during the treatment process.

This, in a nut shell, is a typical clinic shift at WCA. Greet patients new and returning, unpin patients when they are rested and ready to move again, allow time for patients to settle into their treatment environment, check in with and needle patients once they are ready for treatment, and chart a little bit here and there as time permits.

This is one example of community acupuncture in practice. I helped 21 patients this shift. Sometimes you start slow and get busier as the day goes on, other times you start with a full schedule and have cancellations. It is a living breathing healing environment that allows people time to rest and heal from so many different stressors that come up in life. This is a busy and dynamic workplace that gives back in many ways both to the individual acupuncturist, in seeing patients get well and express their appreciation, and to the greater community through providing much needed access to healthcare.

Slowing Down to Speed Up
by Matthew

My road towards becoming a full-time Community Acupuncture practitioner has been long and bumpy, but here I am, and as a few posts have indicated, lots of people are in a place I can definitely relate to.
First off, I think people need to not be so hard on themselves, this is really difficult to get, it seems to me, especially if you haven't been in practice a long time, or even if you have and just haven't been that busy. There are a couple of different obstacles to overcome before you're really comfortable with seeing 40+ patients a week. One of them is timing.

1. Timing

What helped me, and still does if I find I am getting bogged down, is a "self-indulgence" rule: I would look at the clock and give myself 5 minutes, in that time, I could indulge in question asking, palpating, theorizing, etc. All of the mental noise we tend to generate as acupuncturists, but when that time was up, I had to put in needles and walk away. Whatever treatment plan I had devised up to then was what they were gonna get, if some inspiration moved me to a particular point that was not in the plan, sure I'd needle it, but I wouldn't start second guessing or reformulating the basic strategy. Conversely, even if there were a dozen more points I wanted to do, when the 10 minute mark rolled around, that would be time to wrap it up, put in your last two needles and again, walk away. You only spend the time you actually have, and let go of the outcome. Eventually your thinking becomes limited to conclusions you can make with a modicum of information, and the time limit sets the pace for the level of theoretical complexity you can achieve. By slowing down and then completely minimizing the mental process, you actually become faster. I still don't live up to this, but I try.

2. The Confidence Game

This brings us to the next, and probably the biggest, obstacle: confidence. There are three aspects of this, the confidence we have that our treatments work, the confidence that patients have in our treatments, and finally confidence that 90% of the time, 10 minutes is more than enough time.

Confidence in my treatments was easy. I was fortunate enough to barely pay attention in class and instead listened to my wonderful mentors and studied things that are actually expedient to practice (as well as a heapin' helpin' o' big league theory and classics) while in school. I never took anything at face value, if it didn't work, and for me in most cases that meant immediately, it got discarded. Consequently, I studied the meridian therapists, whether they be Japanese, French-Vietnamese or good ol' Dr. Tung (or his theoretical disciple Dr. Tan), and I suggest to anyone looking to build their confidence to start here.

This isn't some anti-TCM screed, just that Meridian Therapy lends itself to a more exploratory approach and all major teachers from these schools believe in instantaneous results--maybe not cure, but some sort of change. When we see these changes manifest right then and there we begin to truly gain confidence that what we are doing is real, concrete and effective. I think many practitioners have rather unhealthy levels of doubt, there will always be some doubt and this medicine has its limitations, but I'm just talking about change--if you felt it, if they felt it, you both know something is happening, this is good, end of story.

I personally used to do A LOT of palpation and interaction with my patients, asking for feedback about points, the effected area (in cases of pain), etc. I still probably do more than the other practitioners here at WCA, but it's part of my style and not necessarily a liability in the timing department. If you work within the limitations (time or otherwise) of this system, there's really no limit to the different styles you can practice.

The real obstacle is letting go of your patient's confidence in your treatments. Here's where the lion's share of doubt creeps in. It used to drive me absolutely crazy when I'd have a patient's neck pain reduced to almost nothing in the chair, and the next week they'd say the treatment didn't change anything. WHAT? You came in here with a 6-7/10, it went down to 1/10 for a couple of hours and you can't see the progress in that!?! Here's the thing: they came back, and most people will come back even if you do absolutely NOTHING to change their condition. You don't have to cure something in one shot, even if you do, it's not required that the patient even realize it. As long as they are coming back, some part of them knows this is a good thing to be doing.

At a certain point I realized almost all of my palpating for ashi points was really to show THEM there was something there, and almost all of my asking for feedback was either trying to get THEM to acknowledge a change, or to try and make the treatment perfect. Patients that expect miracle cures as a matter of course are not the right kind of patients for acupuncture in general, and especially not for community style acupuncture. Treatments don't have to be perfect, now instead of asking for feedback until I run out of time or the symptom disappears, I ask until they feel significantly better, then I do what I'm gonna do, if it has a better effect or not, who cares? Reducing symptoms 50% for any amount of time is plenty for most people to understand that something more than placebo is happening.

Things get ugly when you start assuming that your patients are displeased that you didn't cure them in one treatment, you start to lose ground in your confidence, don't let this happen! YOU are the acupuncturist, managing expectations is not about telling them it won't work like they think it should, it's letting them discover how acupuncture does work. People have all sorts of preconceptions, let them have them and let them play-out naturally, most people simply "get it" after a few treatments. If a patient makes an issue out of how on treatment 3 they aren't able to throw away their crutches, then it's time to simply explain that acupuncture doesn't work that way. They'll usually decide to listen to the expert (you) or they're probably in that "miracle cure" group, and your time and energy are not used wisely in trying to live up to that. It's actually a very small group of patients, and choosing not to play that game is better for BOTH of you in the end.

3. The Devil in the Details

The last obstacle is The Perfect Treatment. Oh! If only I had more time, I could whip-up The Perfect Treatment. Not to beat a dead horse, but any treatment that can be done in 10 minutes and still effects some sort of change IS the perfect treatment. This is very closely related to all or nothing thinking. When patients question the process it's usually either/or thinking at work, ie "either acupuncture works or it doesn't" and consequently we get into the old "either I'm good at acupuncture or I'm not".

Here's where the "frequency of treatments" aspect comes in. It takes time. All healing takes time. If you have a miracle treatment, it's very likely that the patient has already done the majority of the healing before even coming to you. Sometimes they aren't ready and you keep treating them--with absolutely no effect--until they are, then they have that miracle break through. Mostly, though, people get better step-by-step. Most people have been through enough in their lives to understand what it is to heal without any help and therefore instantly recognize how acupuncture facilitates it. Even the most radical healing, surgery, takes time. The recovery from the trauma, that's part and parcel of the process, it's as much of the healing as the cutting. Even "faith" healing requires that the patient be ready for it, and I'll wager even that takes time. So, The Perfect Treatment is really a myth, you just happened to be the right thing at the right time. Recognizing this will set you free in your practice. Every damn treatment where a patient shows up is the perfect treatment!

OK, I've Built It. Now Where the Heck Are They? Some Thoughts on Growing a Patient Base by Lisa

WCA has been open for six years (Good Lord!) and I have had lots of opportunities to reflect on the dynamics of how the schedule book fills up or empties out. Some of those opportunities occurred early on when there was nobody there for me to treat, the phone wasn't ringing, and there was pretty much nothing else for me to think about. It's hard to think about anything else when you are staring at the possibility of failure at uncomfortably close range. As far as I can tell, an empty appointment book is caused by three categories of potential issues, with one general qualification.

Let's get the general qualification out of the way first: life is cyclical. Things change. Things go up and down. If you don't believe me, ask the I Ching. No matter what else is going on, there will be some oscillation of patient numbers in any practice. There will be slow times and peak times. That's just how it is. If you want to eliminate that element of fluctuation, you are going to need to find another dimension of reality to put your practice in.

For those of us who will be staying in this dimension, the question really is -- how slow is slow? How do I arrange things so that "slow" is not an economic crisis? This is where I think the three categories of causes-of-an-empty-appointment-book come in, and they are:

1. Energy (Yours)
2. Ambivalence (Also yours)
3. Structure (which is really a combination of the first two, and still yours.)

The general qualification, that patient numbers will oscillate, has to do with other people's energy, other people's ambivalence, and other people's structure. Practicing medicine, unless you are a veterinarian, means dealing with people, and people are an unreliable lot. If they were more reliable, they would have less need of healers. So your patients' inability to focus their energy, clarify their intentions, resolve their ambivalence, and organize their lives -- everything that leads them to not make appointments with you -- is just what you signed on to deal with when you decided you wanted to be a healer. Hey, nobody said this was a glamorous job (well, actually, some people have kind of implied that, but they are full of ****.)

1. Energy

Okay, back to the categories. Number one: energy. If you are tired, divided, or distracted, you will have fewer patients. If you're VERY tired, divided, or distracted, you will probably have no patients at all. Many new practitioners are very tired at exactly the time when their clinics open -- because they've been doing all the work to get their clinics ready. Or they have just graduated from school. They're tapped out. The only remedy for this is rest. (Hard to do when you are worried about money, I know, but there it is.) If I teach a weekend workshop and try to see patients on Monday morning, I'll be looking at a lot of empty slots. Recently we changed the schedule at WCA so that I don't work Monday mornings anymore -- it was kind of pointless.

Similarly for divided or distracted -- if something else has major claims on your physical, emotional, or mental energy, your patient numbers, or lack thereof, will reflect that. Every year in the fall, Skip's patient numbers take a big dip on Wednesday mornings -- it's as reliable as the almanac. That's because cross-country season starts in the fall, and 2 of our 3 kids have been cross-country runners. Wednesday afternoons are when the meets happen, and Skip goes to all of them, like the very supportive dad he is. On Wednesday morning, his energy is not really in the clinic -- it's already directed toward the Franklin High Cross Country Team. So patients don't show up.

If you're like me, you may not really realize that you are tired, divided, or distracted, until you look at your mysteriously empty schedule. Then you may say, aha.

2. Ambivalence

This is a tough one to talk about -- it's hard to be honest enough without making people angry or frustrated. This is where Somerset Maugham's book <u>The Razor's Edge</u> comes in handy. I read this book because my meditation teacher recommended it, and it's not just because the title comes from the Katha Upanishad; it's because the conclusion of the book is that in life, people basically get whatever it is that they truly want. One reason that you might not be attracting patients is because you don't really want them. Don't scream; let me explain.

This is where some seemingly disparate issues come together. Many students were taught in acupuncture school that doing a good job with patients means doing things that in their heart of hearts they don't really want to do. Furthermore, a lot of patients don't really want you to do them either. But that is a bit of an aside, because what matters here is what you want. If you really believe that to do a good job with a patient, to give him what he really needs, you have to spend an hour talking to him, carefully pore over his medical history, come up with a perfect Zang-Fu diagnosis, do half an hour of Tui Na, and write up a brilliant herbal prescription, all the while fluffing his pillows attentively, do you still want to see him? How about him, his wife, and all their friends and relatives? Really? Do you feel a tiny internal cringe when you think about what it would really mean to do treatments like that over and over? For years? I feel more than a tiny cringe, I feel a wave of exhaustion and hopelessness engulf me when I think about practicing like that. The hopelessness comes from knowing that a whole lot of patients don't really even need all that -- not to mention can't pay for it --but if I really believed that's what a "good treatment" is, I'd feel compelled to do it.

Hello, ambivalence.

It's ironic that some of the people in the acupuncture profession who define what a "good treatment" is are not actually practicing full time. They are teaching in schools, or on the CEU circuit, and they're teaching a mode of practice that is impractical and unsustainable. They're being paid to create standards which they have no intention of upholding themselves -- except sporadically, in the tiny private practices that they don't need to depend on to make their living. Sometimes they sprinkle a little salt in the wound by commenting gravely and sadly on how many acupuncturists burn out over the long term.

Then there's ambivalence part two, which I thought about as I was talking to a new CAN practitioner who was worried about her lack of patients. "The other thing is that there are so many other acupuncturists around here, " she said sadly. "I don't know if I can even break in."

The important thing to remember here is that the patients that you really want are not the patients who would be thinking of going to an acupuncturist. They are not the people who are concerned about their health, who are investigating their options, who are hanging out in natural food stores and surfing the Internet for information about whatever condition they have. Well, you might get a few of those. But they are not your patient base. Your patient base is made up of people who are in pain, who are stressed, who are desperately worried about being able to get better so that they can go back to work, who couldn't care less whether what helps them is "natural", unnatural, or polka dotted with green stripes. They just want to feel better. Those are the people who really need you.

When Michael Smith of NADA called me recently, he waxed poetic about the troubles of our profession, and among them he included the problem of "treating groupies". I wouldn't have thought of it like this, but I thought that was a great term. He mentioned a patient at a student clinic who said she had seen FIFTY SEVEN DIFFERENT ACUPUNCTURISTS. "How can you possibly evaluate a patient like that?" Michael said. "They're too busy evaluating you." When I was in school, this was what I learned too -- that I needed to target the patients who were savvy enough to know that they needed me, who were sophisticated enough to really value my services. What I learned later was that those were the patients whom I was least likely to be able to help -- in part because they weren't really sick, they were mostly bored. "Natural medicine" is a hobby for a certain group of patients; it's a lifestyle accoutrement. It has nothing to do with need, or pain, or really, with medicine. If that is who I thought I was supposed to be treating, my schedule book would be empty too. Because I don't want to be a lifestyle accoutrement, I want to be a healer.

One thing here that you have to know is that building a patient base out of people who really need you does not happen over night. Because they don't know anything about you; they haven't seen 57 people like you and it will take time for them to understand what you have to offer. Once they figure it out, though, they will overwhelm you with their devotion, their goodwill, and their commitment to your practice.

If your schedule book is chronically on the empty side, it's worth doing a really thorough internal inventory of what you think a good treatment is, who you think you are supposed to be treating, and whether, honestly, you really want to do those things and see those people. It's damn hard to manifest work that you don't really like. (Thank you, Somerset Maugham.) To figure out what you do like and what you can do, you may have to spend some serious time and energy de-programming yourself. Think about where you got your ideas about what acupuncture is. Was it from someone who was actually doing acupuncture? How much acupuncture? For how long?

3. Structure

Okay, on to structure. Structure has to do with what happens once you have attracted a patient to your clinic. I learned my big lesson about structure when I was working in my practice pretty much alone (Skip was still paying our mortgage by doing public health.) I had gotten up to a steady 30 patients a week and I couldn't get beyond that. The day that I figured out why, I had one patient waiting for me to treat them, I was trying to schedule another patient for next week, I knew that we had just run out of toilet paper in the bathroom, my landlord was coming in ten minutes to try to fix a problem with our electrical panel, I had a stack of filing that was spilling all over my desk, and the plants needed to be watered -- dead leaves were falling on my pile of filing. And then the phone rang. I picked it up and snarled, "What! What do YOU want!"

That night I begged Ilse, my neighbor, to come in and answer the phones for me. I thought she'd be great at it, and she was -- but it really didn't matter, as she certainly could not have been worse than me.

If the structure of how your clinic handles patients is exhausting for you, you will have trouble attracting patients, because on some level you won't really want to see them. If having patients in your clinic means that you have to do things that you really, really don't want to do -- like, in my case, answering the phone or otherwise multitasking -- you will not attract patients. Not because you don't like doing acupuncture, but because you don't like doing what goes along with doing acupuncture.

For your structure to attract patients to your clinic, the structure itself needs to feel simple, pleasant, and easy both to you and to your patients. Ask yourself -- do you like your structure? Really? Are you expecting too much of yourself or of anyone else? Is it time to ask for help?

Practice, Practice, Practice
by Moses

Throughout my childhood I found myself observing or participating in art classes on a regular basis. For over twenty years my father taught drawing, painting, and color theory at the local art college and in private classes. Many of these classes were held in the evenings and as a young high school student that gave me the opportunity to spend time in town with friends or skateboard before driving 20 miles back to our rural home. Sometimes, though, at the end of one of these evenings, I would hangout in my dad's classroom and, out of interest, participate in some of the class exercises. From these many experiences one particular exercise that my dad taught still stands out in my mind due its mix of challenge, fun, and fright. The exercise is simple. My dad would "loosen up the class and get the creative juices flowing" by asking people to draw or paint a complete picture, with all necessary details, color, and shading, in one minute. Further, students would repeat this exercise ten times in ten minutes and then basically have a small art show at the end to show for their effort.

My dad discovered that when students work in this way they go through most of the same emotions that he goes through to complete any piece of art, just that all of these emotions that come up in the creative process are condensed into one minute. First, students are overwhelmed and a little excited to begin a new project, second, they are scared and frustrated that they have to create a whole piece of art in a short amount of time, third, they are either determined to push through and make it happen or feel stuck from fear of failure and have a very hard time starting the work at all. Fourth, there is the experience of being cut off in the middle of working once the minute is over, which seemed to bring up mixed emotions depending on the individual student.

This intense focus for short periods of time is both potentially emotionally exhausting and eventually, with lots of practice, energizing due to the various emotional walls that come up and are pushed through while making decisions in such quick succession due to the one minute time limit. After the first picture is completed, many students would begin to slow down and take a breath when they suddenly remember that they have to continue with the same process nine more times before the exercise is over. After a few seconds of frantic preparation, students once again go through the whole process of creating a complete picture until the exercise is over. Around the third minute mark I would often notice a kind of meditative hum of focused action throughout the art class.

Once the ten minutes and ten drawings or paintings are complete, there is a collective pause and moment of calm reflection on what just happened. After the paintings are displayed and people start milling about the room there is a mix of pride and embarrassment as people see what they and others created. The sense of pride, however small, gained from decisive action in the midst of time pressure is briefly discussed in class, and students are acknowledged for completing the exercise in whatever form they could.

Art and Community Acupuncture

I could always tell the students that had done the one minute exercise in previous classes because those students were quick to get to work without first going through obvious emotional pause and preparation. Also, students familiar with the exercise tended to have more completed works by the end and more consistently powerful strokes in the images they created. One thing that struck me in these exercises was that some very accomplished artists who completed the exercise had a hard time with it, which I had not anticipated. I suppose it potentially showed that working quickly is not a good fit for all people, or that those unaccustomed to a quick pace would struggle more at first and eventually prevail.

Creating one minute drawings or paintings is similar to providing community acupuncture (CA) treatments in five or ten minute increments because in each discipline the practitioner gets to the creative essence or flow state of an activity by making critical decisions under time pressure. In my experience, this time pressure encourages a clear goal oriented focus coupled with a personalized approach that becomes increasingly more effective and efficient through practice. As you participate in the art class exercise you get more comfortable with developing the structure of your drawing or painting quickly and effectively. It is always a challenging exercise due to the time constraint, yet the results tends to get increasingly bold, clear, goal oriented and powerful in proportion to the students' familiarity with the exercise.

A similar process of refinement through practice happens in practicing CA. Over time a community acupuncture practitioner (CAP) develops efficiency of diagnostic skill and eventually an intake with a new patient becomes shorter due to this refined skill level. CA practitioners assess which questions and orientation information are most relevant to a new patient from how the patient holds themselves, their tone of voice, the level of animation in their bodies, and how they interact with their environment. This refinement of assessment skills is of course true for all types of acupuncturists, yet CA provides a unique venue for quick development of these types of practitioner skills. Treating a high volume of patients each day translates into encountering and pushing through unfamiliar practitioner/ patient experiences often, which in turn forces the CA practitioner to develop his or her communication skills rapidly.

My dad was fond of relating that art was something you had to do in a state of mind where you set your expectations and personal boundaries for expression aside for the moment and just create. When in a purely creative state of mind, one performs in ways one might never believe possible by allowing the experience to happen without getting carried away by judgment or by fear of failure. When you allow yourself to do something without projecting judgment about your ability to achieve that goal, you step into a place of power and efficiently guide your hopes and intentions through your actions as you create.

Your first ever one minute drawing may look anywhere from unrecognizable to OK to great, yet, as you practice over and over again your lines on the canvas or paper become more steady and you develop a confidence and power in your efficiency. As genuine confidence builds the result in your experience is a power and life that begins to show in the images. Eventually, a one minute drawing becomes a relatively smooth and stable endeavor, with natural pacing amid careful efficiency. With practice, you find that you don't need a whole minute to get the basic scene drawn, and that you start filling in more and more details in that same period of time.

In the same way that the impressionist painting style creates a sense of aliveness in the images portrayed, without relying heavily on realist detail, the CA practitioner creates simple yet powerful acupuncture treatments in a short period of time. Impressionism struck a cord with my father. He draws and paints quickly, with determined strokes and when I watch him work I see a blur of lines and movement and then suddenly the energy or impression of the scene or subject emerges. My dad feels comfortable using only enough lines to get the job done and occasionally comments to his students that you can "over-paint" a painting and ruin the effectiveness of portraying the energy of the environment you are looking at through adding excess detail.

Just as my father's art students learned to create impressive works of art in one minute, CA practitioners can learn to treat patients powerfully and efficiently in 5 to 15 minute interactions. Treating patients with this style of acupuncture is a skill that can be developed. It is simply a matter of having a passion for this type of business model and the perseverance to practice, practice, practice. . .

If I Were Going to Start My Own Acupuncture School
by Joseph

Not that I'm really thinking of starting my own school, but if I were. . . one of the introductory first year courses I would require for my students would be to work in a restaurant waiting tables. I believe it's a great training for an acupuncturist, especially if you are going to practice community acupuncture. Besides its practical applications such as fairly flexible schedules, good part-time income for a student and the food benefits, it requires multitasking skills that the new acupunk will need in the community acupuncture setting.

I often think about how similar treating patients as a community acupuncturist is to waiting tables. Instead of turning tables we flip chair covers. (checking for stray needles, not crumbs) Instead of people telling me what they want I figure out what they need. Both jobs require to very quickly determining how to best communicate with patients/patrons effectively. In both scenarios people typically want their check or wake up from their nap at the same time. I usually scan the room to check on each person while they are reclining just as a good waiter/tress will make sure all the needs of their patrons are being met. The waitperson brings food while the acupuncturist checks on comfort by offering an extra blanket or adjusting the chair.

In a busy shift both acupuncturist and waiter lose a sense of time as they are working ("in the face of creativity time becomes meaningless"). There are so many details to consider which require a lot of focus with both occupations. Just as a busy restaurant shift can energize a person, a slow acupuncture shift can equally make a person tired and lethargic. When people are coming and going the energy flows and it's palpable. (Especially the thick "Qi" permeating the acupuncture clinic.)

Often times patients will all show up at the same time. I like to acknowledge each patient so they know I will be with them as soon as I am able. In restaurant lingo when you are very busy (overwhelmed) you are "in the weeds". I can't remember where that expression came from, but that's another story. In the acupuncture clinic when it gets hectic I'll take a deep breath and make sure I am grounded so I can focus completely with each person. I know when I have lots of patients to treat (or to serve) I do my best work because I have to be efficient as well as think with my heart and hands and not as much with my head.

I wonder what my teachers would say about my school with foundational table waiting as part of the acupuncture curriculum? In addition to memorizing point location there would be the experiential requirement of interacting with lots of hungry impatient people. One course could be entitled Table Diagnosis

101. How to handle the….And of course I would have to submit test questions to the NCCAOM. Who knows, it could catch on…Either way, don't forget to tip your waitperson.

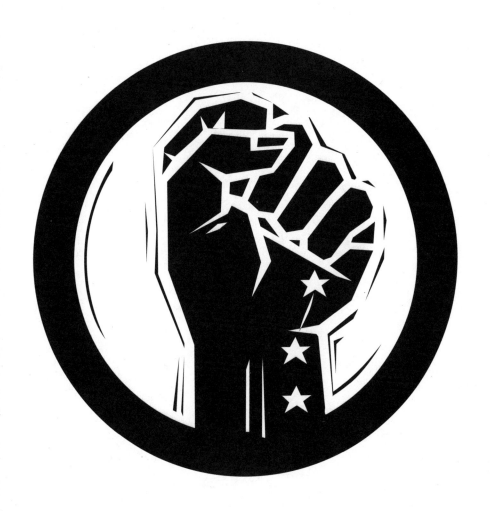

Part Five: Health Care Reform and Noodles

Recently our clinic had the opportunity to host one of the Health Care Community Discussions (otherwise known as "health care house parties") sponsored by the Health Policy Transition Team of the incoming Obama administration. The Transition Team provided a moderator's packet with a set of questions, and asked for a "group statement" at the end. Here is the group statement that we came up with:

> First, we want to offer a huge enthusiastic thank you to the Health Policy Transition Team. We began our discussion with pretty much everyone saying that we were somewhat stunned by the fact that the government actually wanted to know what we think about health care. We were surprised to be asked, to be acknowledged, to be invited into the conversation. Simply being INCLUDED in a national discussion about health policy seemed like a very big deal to us. After spending two hours together talking about issues that matter enormously to all of us, we felt as if we had somehow participated in history.
>
> Through the course of the discussion we discovered a remarkable unity amongst ourselves. There are a number of core points that, although they were raised by different people, resonated deeply with everyone.
>
> The first point was that though we appreciated the questions offered as guidelines for the discussion, we needed to take our discussion beyond the parameters of the questions. Beginning with the first question of what is wrong with health care in America, we arrived pretty quickly at a consensus that the system is so broken and so unresponsive to our needs and the needs or our families, that what we really need is a complete paradigm shift. The system needs more than repairs; we think its foundations are askew.

We agreed that health care is a public need rather than an individual need, not unlike the need for roads, a postal service, or basic education. Individuals should not be as responsible as they are for figuring out how to make health care happen for themselves and their families, any more than individuals should be responsible for figuring out how to make the roads work before they can drive on them, or make the postal service work before they can mail a letter, or make the education system work before they can send their children to school. There are so many national systems that really do work; why can't health care be another one?

We also felt strongly that the health care system in its current state is clearly NOT FOR US. It is not designed to benefit or help us. Who is it for? Who does it benefit? We suspect that the answer is big corporations, because none of us know any individuals who feel that the health care system really meets their needs. It's bureaucratic, disempowering, overwhelming, confusing, and frustrating in more ways than we can list.

We all agreed that the profit motive for health care has got to be removed. Medicine should not be a lucrative practice. We favor salaries that are livable for health care providers, but we do not think the reward for being involved in health care should be financial. (We had two nurses and four licensed acupuncturists in our group.) Lower salaries would probably translate to a greater number of jobs. Similarly, the litigious aspect of the health system needs to be reined in; there should be no profit motive for lawyers. (We had a lawyer in our group.)

We decided together that we need to "redefine the discourse". Even the questions you offered us as guidelines for the discussion were couched in the status quo. Prevention, for example, means more to us than just early detection of disease. Health is more than the absence of illness.

The idea of "health insurance" does not really make sense to us. As responsible adults, we have car insurance, we have home insurance, we understand how insurance works. Car insurance and home insurance work as a concept because most of us are not going to total our cars or have our roofs cave in. You get insurance with the expectation that it is unlikely that something will go so badly wrong that you will need to use it. But human bodies are not like cars or houses; all of us are definitely going to have something go wrong with us someday. All of us are going to die. You can't base health care on a system that presumes you shouldn't need to use it.

We agreed that we do not actually want "health insurance". We want "health assurance". We want to know that we will get the care we need, when we need it. We understand our own responsibility for making our lives as healthy as possible, but we want to know that there is a larger system to help us, a system that is based on the public good rather than individual profit. We do not expect to precisely fulfill every one of our individual preferences; we are prepared to compromise and adjust as long as we know that the point of the system is to take care of people. We believe that there should be an assurance of basic services for everyone.

All of us in our discussion group are either staff or patients of Working Class Acupuncture, an acupuncture clinic that treats over 400 people a week, located in a "marginal" neighborhood in Northeast Portland. We all agreed that we wished the whole health care system was more like WCA, which has a community based business model. We all feel invested in and empowered by our clinic; we feel that it represents the concerns of working class people around health care. We loved the experience of having this discussion with each other, of creating and sharing a collective vision. We all left feeling uplifted and connected to each other in a new way, so thank you again for encouraging us to participate in this process.

This statement does a good job, we think, of reflecting the overall perspective on health care reform of our little community of WCA staff and patients. It does not address, however, the specific issue of how acupuncture relates to health care reform. And we cannot address that without asking what kind of reform acupuncture in America needs, itself.

Nobody Owns Acupuncture: Licensing, Classism, and Turf Warfare

The short answer to that question is: like other forms of health care, the profit motive in acupuncture has got to go. Nobody owns acupuncture; people should be able to make a living by doing it, because it is something society needs, but acupuncture is not something that is meant to make anybody rich. Also, since nobody owns acupuncture, all sorts of people besides licensed acupuncturists ought to be able to legally practice it, because it is so safe and so noninvasive.

Historically, acupuncturists had to fight to be able to practice legally, without being supervised by a physician. Legal practice was made possible by the passage of laws in most states that created independent licensure for acupuncturists. From our perspective, the point of licensing laws is to make acupuncture available to as many people as possible, rather than keeping it underground. Unfortunately, the next step after licensing laws for many acupuncturists was turf warfare: trying to make sure that nobody else could practice acupuncture except licensed acupuncturists. Many acupuncture associations consider their primary goal to be the defense of their professional turf against incursions by chiropractors, osteopaths, physical therapists, massage therapists, and anyone else who has the temerity to believe that they might be able to use an acupuncture needle without enduring three to four years of memorizing Chinese medical theory. Many acupuncturists consider NADA's Acupuncture Detoxification Specialists to be adversaries as well, since a NADA ADS can -- horror of horrors -- put needles in ears with only 70 hours of training.

Licensed acupuncturists who hold this territorial perspective would doubtless consider this book to be guilty of gross oversimplification on every level, since they usually justify turf warfare on the basis that acupuncture is such a complex system of medicine that it can only be safely practiced by extremely specialized professionals. Most likely none of those people are reading this paragraph, however, since having to read over and over about how much acupuncture is like noodles in the first part of this book would have induced death by apoplexy much earlier on in their reading experience. Alas, we feel very little sympathy. They never liked us anyway, and we treat a lot more patients than they do.

Since everyone who has contributed to this book is a licensed acupuncturist, why, you might be wondering, are we such traitors to our own kind? It's because we see turf warfare as class warfare, and you can probably guess whose side we are on when it comes to class warfare. Although practitioners of turf warfare claim that they are only trying to protect the public, what they are most concerned with is really their own status. By limiting who can practice acupuncture, they hope to define the licensed acupuncturist as yet another upper middle class professional. This goes along with defining suitable professional compensation, which in turn leads to charging $100 and up for an acupuncture treatment because physical therapists charge $100 and up for a session. Turf warfare is about keeping up with the Joneses -- that is, the Dr. Joneses. The collateral damage to patients from turf warfare by raising the cost of acupuncture and limiting the number of practitioners never seems to enter the discussion.

Our desire in practicing acupuncture is not to enter the ranks of the upper middle class. Our desire is to take care of our own communities, and it is clear to us that what our communities need is lots of simple, inexpensive acupuncture. We look forward to the day that acupuncture is so cheap that no one wants to fight over it anymore, and the people who need it most can just have as much of it as they want. Perhaps this is why we are so often accused by other licensed acupuncturists of "devaluing the profession"?

What acupuncturists have typically contributed to the discussion about health care reform are demands that they receive more recognition and better compensation -- in short, that they should be able to bill insurance companies at a par with physical therapists, chiropractors, etc., because licensed acupuncturists are such wonderful holistic healers and everybody needs us. (If we are such wonderful holistic healers and everybody needs us, why are we not taking responsibility for the fact that almost no one can afford us?) When the discussion about single payer health care comes up, what most acupuncturists want to talk about is getting their piece of the pie, as long as that piece comes with a $100 per treatment price tag.

We feel a need to radically redefine this particular discourse.

Acupuncture is so old, and so simple, and so flexible, that nobody can possess or control it. Acupuncture has come down to us in the present as a gift from the past; it's ridiculous to act as if we are entitled to anything. The only question worth asking is, what would Sun Simiao do in the midst of a health care crisis? You know, that 6th century guy who talked about how a great practitioner "should not desire anything and should ignore all consequences"?

Beyond Professionalism, Toward Usefulness

No profession is an end in itself. Medical professions, in particular, depend on a foundation of altruism for their integrity. The point is to give, not to take; in terms of acupuncture, the point is to provide a means for acupuncture to reach as many people as possible. If you are going to make acupuncture your vocation, it is your responsibility to share acupuncture rather than to hoard it. The model created by NADA is a shining example of sharing rather than hoarding; it's a good example to look at as we consider the reform of acupuncture in America.

The model of NADA suggests that we should think about where acupuncture is needed before we think about who provides it. Once we identify where acupuncture is needed, we can come up with creative, simple, elegant ways to put it there. This goes along with transforming the basic unit of acupuncture treatment. Instead of having one cubicle, one table, one patient, and one acupuncture professional with a big ego and lots of letters behind his or her name -- which is a cumbersome, expensive unit -- we could have an efficient, inexpensive unit, consisting of one community room, multiple comfortable places to rest, and multiple patients comfortably resting, with needles that were put there by someone who knew what he or she was doing. Knowing what you are doing with acupuncture can happen in, oh, 70 hours or so.

These community acupuncture treatment units could provide acupuncture efficiently and inexpensively in all sorts of settings: not only substance abuse treatment programs but hospitals, nursing homes, urgent care facilities, doctors' offices, senior centers, and community centers. Anyone who is trained and licensed to give injections or do sutures could learn to use a few simple acupuncture protocols in a matter of weeks -- and could relieve an enormous amount of suffering. For example, the NADA auricular protocol itself is effective not only for the symptoms of drug and alcohol detox but also for the relief of pain and stress in general. Because these community acupuncture units need so little to function: a quiet room, comfortable places for patients to rest, needles that cost a few cents each, and a person to put them in who knows how to do it -- they could easily become financially self-supporting by using patient fees on a sliding scale similar to ours. Which would mean that hospitals, nursing homes, urgent care facilities, doctors' offices, senior centers, and community centers could provide acupuncture at virtually no cost to themselves. You can see by reviewing Parts Two and Three of this book how easy this would be to accomplish.

Instead of failing to become the basis for yet another upper middle class profession -- and acupuncture is failing at this, because almost no one can afford it -- acupuncture could succeed wildly as a humble, ubiquitous, miraculous modality that nobody owns and everybody uses. Imagine the impact of acupuncture seeping into every corner of our dysfunctional health care system: quietly relieving pain without pharmaceuticals, reducing stress without psychotherapy, inexorably changing the way people think about health and illness by providing an ongoing testimonial to people's ability to heal themselves. Acupuncture doesn't need upper middle class professionals, and upper middle class professionals should not be permitted to hijack acupuncture.

What the Future Could Look Like...

The first step toward realizing acupuncture's enormous potential usefulness is simply to make a distinction between the theory and practice of acupuncture. It would be nice if Chinese medical theory were something that people could study in undergraduate liberal arts programs as a subject that is interesting for its own sake, like pre-Socratic philosophy or medieval French poetry, but which also comes with limited expectations of being able to apply it out in the world. Many people end up becoming acupuncturists primarily because they find Chinese medical theory fascinating, not because they want to help people; there should be other ways to scratch that particular itch. An undergraduate college which added a certificate program in Chinese medical theory would immediately attract many students. (Hint, hint.)

Similarly, nursing schools should be able to add a certificate program in the clinical practice of acupuncture. The bulk of what we do in our clinic could be taught to a nurse in about three months. The same goes for physician assistants, physical therapists, midwives, and anyone else who both takes care of patients and can do injections or sutures. Learning to put in acupuncture needles is significantly less difficult than learning to do injections or sutures, because the needles in question are so much smaller and can be inserted at such a shallow depth. Any of these people could potentially begin to practice community acupuncture a few hours a week within the context of their current jobs, thus providing acupuncture to dozens of patients.

As for the inevitable argument that having a lot of non-acupuncturists using acupuncture protocols is going to result in second-rate treatments, acupuncture not being used to its full potential, etc. -- oh, please. Given what acupuncture's full potential is, using even a fraction of it could make life infinitely better for millions of people. "Second rate" acupuncture could still work miracles. And any acupuncture that patients can actually have is going to be superior to the acupuncture that patients can't actually have, because they can't afford it. Any acupuncture is preferable to no acupuncture. As Voltaire wrote, the perfect is the enemy of the good. (He also wrote: every man is guilty of all the good he did not do.)

And what about the role of the licensed acupuncturist? The irony is that while conventional acupuncturists are seeking to make acupuncture into the foundation for a lucrative, upper middle class profession, what they have created is a situation in which acupuncture is, for many of them, nothing more than an outrageously expensive hobby. A master's degree in acupuncture is currently the functional equivalent of a Ming vase: it costs the earth, and most of the time, all you can really do with it is to admire it. What acupuncture could be instead is a solid lower middle class occupation that is simultaneously creative and satisfying.

A good beginning would be for everyone to understand that, if you are not a health care professional already, you could become a competent, effective licensed acupuncturist in about 18 months with the appropriate kind of education. The appropriate kind of education would be something like a trade school that focused on practical skills and taught acupuncture alone, rather than acupuncture plus Chinese herbs and Tui Na massage and the rest of the Chinese medical kitchen sink that most American schools throw at their students. The reason that we don't have this kind of education right now is that acupuncture schools and acupuncture regulatory agencies were able to persuade many people that licensed acupuncturists should be something more than "mere technicians". This is a good example of classism in action, because the truth is that a well trained technician is much more use to society than an overeducated theorist who rarely or never applies what he learned -- particularly when what we are talking about is the ability to relieve suffering. A whole lot of us would be proud to be called acupuncture technicians, if it meant we were of use to our communities.

Making acupuncture education much shorter and much cheaper would also go a long way towards diversifying the acupuncturist population. We need more acupuncturists who are not white and upper middle class themselves. Our clinic is located in one of the largest, poorest, most ethnically diverse neighborhoods in Portland. Cully neighborhood has one of the lowest ratios of people to parks and one of the highest ratios of taverns to people. Acupuncturists often lament the fact that Portland is "saturated" with acupuncturists -- but we have always been the only acupuncture clinic in Cully, compared to dozens of acupuncturists concentrated in the wealthier neighborhoods of Portland. We are also the largest acupuncture clinic in the state (and possibly the whole country) that is not attached to a school. (Oh, the irony, that the largest free-standing acupuncture clinic in the country is possibly in Cully, with all the taverns and the trailer parks.) There could be hundreds more clinics like ours in neighborhoods like ours, but it would help a lot if they too were owned by acupuncturists who live in and love those neighborhoods, and who identify with their neighbors.

Acupuncture as a solid lower middle class occupation could create tens of thousands of jobs, because it is needed everywhere. Even if legions of nurses and physical therapists and physician assistants begin practicing acupuncture as part of their jobs, the demand for acupuncture would only rise as people began to truly understand what it can do. We like to say that we want to compete with the taverns in Cully, not with other acupuncturists or with doctors. We want to provide not just a medical treatment, but a place for people to escape their troubles and their stress.

The role for licensed acupuncturists in health care reform should be the same as their role in the community acupuncture revolution: to lead the movement to share acupuncture with America. In many NADA programs, a licensed acupuncturist supervises multiple Acupuncture Detoxification Specialists, thus making it possible for hundreds of people to get treatment -- far more than any individual acupuncturist could ever help. Licensed acupuncturists could have a similar role with other health care providers who are learning to offer community acupuncture: instructing, coaching, providing ongoing support, so that their expertise reaches far beyond their own practices. Licensed acupuncturists who love Chinese medical theory could put their brains to use by devising ever more simple and elegant acupuncture protocols based on the Chinese classics. Sharing acupuncture rather than hoarding it opens up infinite possibilities for being useful. Doesn't that seem like what Sun Simiao would do?

Community Acupuncture IS Health Care Reform . . .

. . . because it is inclusive. By making the same service available to people with different financial resources, community acupuncture breaks down the barriers of classism in health care.

. . . because it is low-tech and low-cost. MRIs and CAT scans certainly have their place in health care, but our growing dependence on expensive technologies is part of what is driving up costs. Community acupuncture reverses this trend.

. . . because it is preventative. Community acupuncture can precisely target the intersection of stress and disease, a zone that the big guns of conventional medicine miss by a mile. When acupuncture is cheap enough for patients to use in unlimited quantities, no one has to wait to get sick in order to use it.

. . . because for at least some patients, it can reduce their dependence on Big Pharma. Not everyone can use acupuncture to get off their medications, but when it comes to painkillers, sleep aids, and anti-anxiety drugs, acupuncture is worth trying as a substitute.

. . . because it does not require the approval or the participation of Big Insurance. A community acupuncture clinic depends on the support of its local community, not on a distant, enormous, for-profit corporation.

. . . because it is easy to understand and easy to use. Patients do not have to wade through a maze of bureaucracy to get care.

. . . because it creates jobs rather than profits.

. . . because it breaks down the isolation that is rampant not only in health care, but throughout American culture.

. . . because it is radically transparent and radically simple. Acupuncture depends so much on the internal resources of the patient and so little on external props that it's basically function without form -- a nice change from health care that is form without function. All acupuncture is, is what it does. And all it needs are needles, cotton balls and stillness.

. . . and finally, because it does not need the government or anyone else to fund it. If community acupuncture were readily available, it could save the health care system enormous sums of money by preventing the need for hospitalizations, surgeries, and medication. It would be wonderful if the government recognized this potential -- but even if it doesn't, community acupuncture will continue to grow exponentially. Community acupuncture is truly a grassroots movement, and it flourishes outside of all existing systems. All that community acupuncture needs is more patients and more practitioners who are willing to try it and then apply it in their communities as we have applied it in ours. It is our hope that this book will help reach these people. Thank you for reading it.

Appendix A: Handling Needles

Here's a brief overview of how we handle and insert acupuncture needles.

Opening the Needle Pack

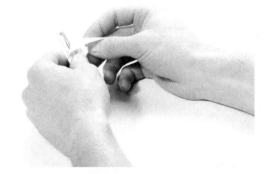

The needles we use at Working Class Acupuncture come in packs of 10. This cuts down on waste, and is much faster once you get the hang of handling more than one needle at a time. When opening a new pack of needles, we open the thick "handle" end of the packet, peeling the paper about halfway down so that the pack itself serves as a clean holder.

Removing the Needle

We pull each needle out by its handle. When holding needles, we are careful to not touch the thin wire "shaft" of the needle, as this is the part that breaks the skin of the patient, and we want to avoid any possible contamination.

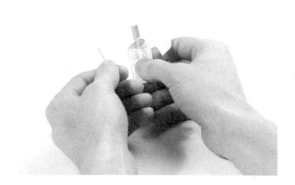

Loading the Guide Tube

Each pack also has a single "guide tube", we use a new tube for each patient, again to avoid possible contamination. Guide tubes help to make the insertion of the needle as painless as possible by giving the thin needles something solid to support them. We hold the tube in one hand and insert the handle end of the needle with the other.

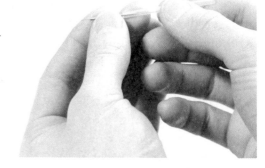

Holding the Needle Ready

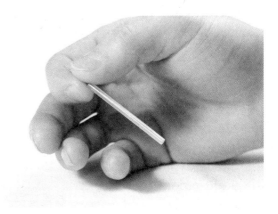

Once the needle is in the guide tube, we tip the tube up, so that the needle slides completely into the tube. Using the pad of our finger, we stop the needle from slipping out. Then, we slowly make more space so that the handle can come out the other side. With the thumb and index finger we pinch the handle down against the tube to hold it in place. We make sure that the sharp tip of the needle is completely inside of the guide tube, as we do not want the tip to come into contact with anything.

Placing the Needle

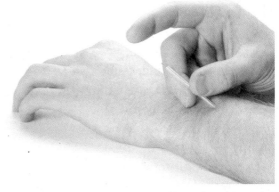

We place the tube on the skin where we located the acupuncture point. Then we let go of the handle with the thumb and finger to allow the needle to slide down, and the sharp tip touch the skin. Holding the tube with the middle finger and thumb, the index finger is kept free. We want a small amount of the handle to be above the edge of the guide tube.

Inserting the Needle

We then press, with a firm but fluid motion, on the handle of the needle until it is even with the edge of the guide tube. This forces the tip to break the skin. The needle is now in place. There are various techniques of insertion; we recommend 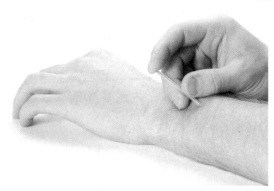 a nice even pace: neither overly fast nor overly slow. There is no need for a forceful "tap" or "flick", smooth technique is more important for the comfort of the patient.

Removing the Guide Tube

Once the needle is in, we simply pull the guide tube away. The needle is not very deep at this point, so some care is needed to avoid pulling it out with the tube. We save the tube for the next point, until we are done with 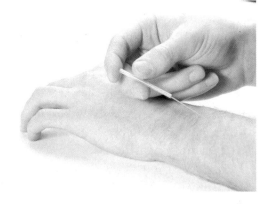 the patient, then discard it. When we come to a new patient, we start with a fresh tube.

Adjusting the Needle

Once the tube is out of the way, we can adjust the depth, and to a certain extent the angle, of the needle. There are myriad, and often contradictory, schools of thought regarding all aspects of needle placement. In our experience, the differences are clinically miniscule, so we recommend people experiment and find what works best for them individually.

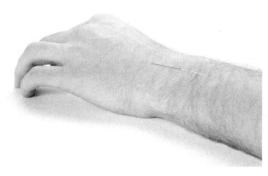

Now do you see why we are suggesting that nurses should be able to practice acupuncture? Anyone who is licensed to do injections can learn how to do this in almost no time at all.

Appendix B: Patient Welcome Letter

Welcome to Our Community!

Please take a minute to read this introduction to our clinic and to our community. We are delighted that you are interested in joining us!

What is different about the WCA clinic?

We treat in a community setting

Most US acupuncturists treat patients on tables in individual cubicles. This is not traditional in Asia, where acupuncture usually occurs in a community setting. In our clinic we primarily use recliners, clustered in groups in a large, quiet, soothing space. Treating patients in a community setting has many benefits: it's easy for friends and family members to come in for treatment together; many patients find it comforting; and a collective energetic field becomes established which actually makes individual treatments more powerful. In some styles of acupuncture, the needles are removed after only a few minutes or after a half hour at most. The style of acupuncture we practice at WCA allows patients to keep their needles in as long as they want, and the "right" amount of time varies from patient to patient. Most people learn after a few treatments when they feel "done"; this can take from twenty minutes to a couple of hours! Many people fall asleep, and wake feeling refreshed.

We have a sliding scale

Most US acupuncturists also see only one patient per hour and charge $65 to $175 per treatment. They tend to spend a long time talking with each patient, going over medical records, asking many questions. We don't. The only way that we at WCA can make acupuncture affordable and still make a living ourselves is to streamline our treatments and see multiple patients in an hour, so we have returned to the traditional approach; instead of asking you lots of questions, we rely on pulse diagnosis to decide how to treat you. This is exactly how acupuncture is practiced traditionally in Asia -- many patients per hour and very little talking.

Please see the enclosed form that explains our sliding scale. Because we have a sliding scale, we cannot do insurance billing (that's the insurance companies' rule). If you have insurance that covers acupuncture, we'll be happy to give you a payment receipt, and you can submit it; that's OK with the insurance companies.

Our Commitment to You

We want to make it possible for you to receive acupuncture regularly enough and long enough to get better and stay better. We want our community to be welcoming to all different kinds of people. We want to give you the tools to take care of your own health so that you will not need to rely on corporations like Big Insurance or Big Pharmaceuticals for costly, high-tech interventions. We will provide a safe environment with skilled practitioners.

What We Need From You

Responsibility

WCA does not provide primary care medicine! Acupuncture is a wonderful complement to Western medicine, but it is not a substitute for it. If you think you have a problem that is not "garden variety" (meaning, you are worried that you might have a serious infection, a malignant growth, or an injury that won't heal), or if you want someone knowledgeable to go over the details of your medical history with you, you need to see a primary care physician (ND, MD, or DO). We can provide some excellent, affordable referrals, even if you have no insurance coverage. But you cannot expect us to diagnose and treat something really serious. We can provide complimentary care for conditions which require a physician's attention -- for instance, we often treat patients for the side effects of chemotherapy. But we need you to take responsibility for your own health.

WCA does not receive grants, state or federal money, or insurance reimbursement. WCA exists because patients pay for their treatments – it a sustainable community business model.

Flexibility

The community setting requires some flexibility from you. For instance, many patients have a favorite recliner. When we are busy, someone may be sitting in yours. Similarly, we have a few patients who snore. Other patients who dislike snoring bring earplugs to their treatments. We are grateful for this! Some of our patients even bring favorite pillows or blankets from home with them, because they prefer theirs to ours. That's fine with us. Basically, we need you to participate in making yourself comfortable in the community room before we arrive to treat you.

In terms of how long you want to stay -- tell the receptionist, when you check in, if you need to be somewhere at a certain time! If you want to be unpinned at a specific time, ask her to make a note and give it to the acupuncturist. We'll make sure you're out on time. In general, if you feel done, open your eyes and give us a meaningful look -- if your eyes are closed, we think you're asleep and we won't wake you up.

Community-Mindedness

The soothing atmosphere in our clinic exists because all of our patients create it by relaxing together. We appreciate everyone's presence! This kind of collective stillness is a rare and precious thing in our rushed and busy society. Maintaining this reservoir of calm requires that no one talk very much in the clinic space. If you would like to speak to a practitioner one-on-one at any length, please let us know. If you want to have a substantial conversation, we will probably need to schedule that separately and might need to do it by phone.

Part of our success is that our patients learn the "routine" and take on a lot of responsibility for the appointments. Re-scheduling and making payment happens at the front desk BEFORE each treatment, so you can relax and enjoy treatment. Please take all personal belongings, (bags, shoes, etc.) with you back into the treatment room. And of course, please turn off your cell phone.

Commitment

Acupuncture is a PROCESS. It is very rare for any acupuncturist to be able to resolve a problem with one treatment. In China, a typical treatment protocol for a chronic condition could be acupuncture every other day for three months! Most of our patients don't need that much acupuncture, but virtually every patient requires a course of treatment, rather than a single treatment, in order to get what they want from acupuncture.

One big reason that we are able to keep our prices so low is because of the extraordinary amount of marketing our patients do on our behalf -- we don't have to advertise. We cannot express how grateful we are for this. Our patients are such effective marketers because they have first-hand experience of how well acupuncture works. All of our satisfied patients basically made a commitment to a course of treatment.

On your first visit, your acupuncturist will suggest a course of treatment, which can be anything from "we'd like to see you once a week for six weeks" to "we'd really like to see you every day for the next four days". This suggestion is based on our experience with treating different kinds of conditions. If you don't come in often enough or long enough, acupuncture probably won't work for you. The purpose of our sliding scale is to help you make that commitment. If you have questions about how long it will take to see results, please ask us, or if you think you need to adjust your treatment plan, please let us know. We need you to commit to the process of treatment in order to get good results.

And, last, but not least….enjoy the space. We do, and hope that Working Class Acupuncture can be an important part of your community. Thank you,

Working Class Acupuncture Staff

Notes

Introduction

1 Joel Rose, "Poor Man's Prick", <u>Good</u> Magazine, November/December 2008

Part One: Acupuncture is Like Noodles

1 Paul Unschuld, <u>Medical Ethics in Imperial China, A Study in Historical Anthropology</u>, copyright 1979 University of California Press, Berkeley, CA
2 Betsy Leondar-Wright, "Working Definitions", <u>Class Matters</u> website. Online. Internet. copyright 2004-2009, http://www.classmatters.org
3 http://pubdb3.census.gov/macro/032008/hhinc/new05_000.htm Online. Internet.
4 Betsy Leondar-Wright, "Are There Class Cultures?" <u>Class Matters</u> website. Online. Internet. copyright 2004-2009, http://www.classmatters.org
5 Thanks to Ruby K. Payne, Ph. D., for the idea of comparing similar social experiences across different classes. <u>Crossing the Tracks for Love: What to Do When You and Your Partner Grew Up in Different Worlds</u>, Ruby K. Payne, copyright 2005 by aha! Process Inc.

Part Two: Welcome to Our Kitchen

1 Zhang Yu Huan and Ken Rose, <u>Who Can Ride the Dragon? An Exploration of the Cultural Roots of Traditional Chinese Medicine</u>, copyright 1995-1999, Paradigm Publications
2 Zhang Yu Huan and Ken Rose, <u>A Brief History of Qi</u>, copyright 2001, Paradigm Publications
3 Michael Pollan, "Unhappy Meals", New York Times, January 28, 2007
4 Zhang Yu Huan and Ken Rose, <u>Who Can Ride the Dragon? An Exploration of the Cultural Roots of Traditional Chinese Medicine</u>, copyright 1995-1999, Paradigm Publications
5 Miram Lee, <u>Insights of a Senior Acupuncturist</u>, copyright 1992, Blue Poppy Press

6 Skip Van Meter, Jingei Pulse Diagnosis DVD, copyright 2007
7 Miram Lee, Insights of a Senior Acupuncturist, copyright 1992, Blue Poppy Press
8 Don't tell us we never tried to bring unity to a fractured profession.
9 If, like lots of acupuncturists, you can't stand not knowing the theory, get our DVD and watch it: Skip Van Meter, Jingei Pulse Diagnosis DVD, copyright 2007
10 Richard Tan and Stephen Rush, Twelve and Twelve in Acupuncture, copyright 1991;
Richard Tan and Stephen Rush, Twenty-Four More in Acupuncture, copyright 1994
11 We do think Master Tung is neat, and interesting, and effective, and we recommend his books. James Maher, trans. and ed., Advanced Tung Style Acupuncture: the Dao Ma Needling Technique of Master Tung Ching-Chang, , copyright 2005
12 Lisa Rohleder, The Remedy: Integrating Acupuncture Into American Healthcare, copyright 2006

Part Three: Welcome to Our Dining Room (and Our Systems)

1 Muhammad Yunus, Creating A World Without Poverty: Social Business and the Future of Capitalism, copyright 2007, Public Affairs, New York, New York, pgs. 21-40
2 Ibid, pg. 54
3 Ibid, pg. 241

Bibliography

Dan Bensky and John O'Connor, trans. and ed., Acupuncture: A Comprehensive Text, Shanghai College of Traditional Medicine, ,copyright 1981, Eastland Press, Seattle

Matthew D. Bauer, The Healing Power of Acupressure and Acupuncture, copyright 2005, the Penguin Group, New York

Zhang Yu Huan and Ken Rose, A Brief History of Qi, , copyright 2001, Paradigm Publications, Brookline

Zhang Yu Huan and Ken Rose, Who Can Ride the Dragon? An Exploration of the Cultural Roots of Traditional Chinese Medicine, copyright 1995-1999, Paradigm Publications, Brookline

Betsy Leondar-Wright, Class Matters website, copyright 2004-2009, http://www.classmatters.org

James Maher, trans. and ed., Advanced Tung Style Acupuncture: the Dao Ma Needling Technique of Master Tung Ching-Chang, , copyright 2005

Ruby K. Payne, Ph.D, Crossing the Tracks for Love: What to Do When You and Your Partner Grew Up in Different Worlds, copyright 2005 , aha! Process Inc.

Michael Pollan, "Unhappy Meals", New York Times, January 28, 2007

Lisa Rohleder, The Remedy: Integrating Acupuncture into American Healthcare, copyright 2006

Joel Rose, "Poor Man's Prick", Good Magazine, November/December 2008

Richard Tan and Stephen Rush, Twelve and Twelve in Acupuncture, copyright 1991

Richard Tan and Stephen Rush, Twenty-Four More in Acupuncture, copyright 1994

Richard Tan, Acupuncture 1,2,3, copyright 2007

Paul Unschuld, Medical Ethics in Imperial China: a Study in Historical Anthropology, copyright 1979 University of California Press, Berkeley

U. S. Census Bureau, "Current Population Survey", http://pubdb3.census.gov/macro/032008/hhinc/new05_000.htm

Muhammad Yunus, Creating a World Without Poverty: Social Business and the Future of Capitalism, copyright 2007, Public Affairs, New York

Acknowledgments

Many people were very helpful in the creation of this book. In no particular order, they are:

Moses Cooper and Matt Gulbranson, for illustrations, editing, graphic design, and attention in general to both details and esthetics;

All of the staff of WCA, receptionists and acupuncturists, for keeping the clinic humming along, seven days a week, in all kinds of weather, and for making the vision a reality;

Joseph Goldfedder, Ann Mongeau, Andy Wegman, Larry Gatti, Korben Perry, Tatyana Ryevzina, Michael Lium-Hall, Lumiel Kim-Hammerich, Cris Monteiro, Nora Madden, and other acupuncturists of the Community Acupuncture Network for endless conversations, online and off, about how to explain exactly what it is we're trying to do;

NADA and Michael Smith, for inspiration and encouragement;

Michael McCoy, for making us think (not to mention also making CAN);

Susan Glosser, for explaining ISBNs and presses;

And Lupine Hudson and Skip Van Meter; they know why.